The Cardiovascular System

Katie

£2.50

Penguin Library of Nursing

General Editor
Michael Bowman

The Cardiovascular System
The Digestive System
The Endocrine System
The Female Reproductive System
The Neuromuscular System
The Respiratory System
The Skeletal System
The Urological System
The Special Senses

The Penguin Library of Nursing Series was created by
Penguin Education and is published by Churchill Livingstone.

P. P. Turner

The Cardiovascular System

Churchill Livingstone

CHURCHILL LIVINGSTONE
Medical Division of Longman Group Limited

Distributed in the United States of America by
Longman Inc., 19 West 44th Street, New York,
N.Y. 10036 and by associated companies,
branches and representatives throughout
the world.

First Edition 1976
Reprinted 1979

ISBN 0 443 01526 0

Printed in Great Britain by
Fletcher & Son Ltd, Norwich

Contents

Editorial foreword

Nursing has undergone considerable change during the past decade. There have been many developments in medical science and technology, and nursing education must keep pace with these changes, not merely in principle, but in terms of the nurse's attitude and approach. These changes primarily stem from the move towards caring for the patient in the context of his entire personality – the concept of total patient care. This concept was originally underlined in the 1962 Experimental Syllabus of Training and has subsequently been mirrored with greater emphasis in the 1969 Syllabus.

The education of the nurse, as voiced nationally and professionally in this decade, has merited prominence; this is certainly underlined in the recent *Report of the Committee on Nursing* (Briggs). It now appears likely that the once rather mythical education of the nurse is now approaching reality and fulfilment. For too long there has been conflict between the service needs of the hospital and the education of the nurse.

These require effective marriage if student satisfaction and general job satisfaction of the officers concerned and, perhaps most important of all, good patient care are all to be achieved. It is hoped that this series of textbooks will go some way towards helping students achieve a better understanding, in a more interesting way, of what this concept of total patient care is all about.

The series consists of nine books; together, these books make up an integrated whole, although each can be used in isolation. Each book embraces developmental embryology, applied anatomy and physiology, pathology, treatment, nursing care, social aspects and rehabilitation of the patient. In addition, each book contains a comprehensive list of further reading for the nurse.

It is hoped that students will find much pleasure in reading these books.

Michael Bowman
Principal, Education Division, Hendon Training School
Examiner to the General Nursing Council for England and Wales

Preface

I consider it a privilege to have been invited to contribute a volume on cardiovascular disease to the Penguin Library of Nursing. In these days of highly specialized nursing in special intensive care areas, much more is demanded of the nurse than was many years ago. At one time many people believed that nurses' training was aimed at producing second-class doctors instead of first-class nurses, but now most realize that the nurse needs a great deal of complex medical knowledge and fundamental understanding if she is to carry out her task intelligently and ably, getting satisfaction from knowing she is doing it well. Human kindness and sympathy is still the basis of good nursing but a great deal of technical skill and know-how is also essential.

It is hoped that, by integrating normal development, anatomy and physiology with pathological processes, social circumstances and resultant disease, the background is set for a proper understanding of treatment, nursing and possible preventive measures thus making sense of the phrase 'total patient care'!

Coronary Care Units have shown us, if we had not already known, the importance of the nurse today. She makes the observations on which treatment is based and indeed must be trained to initiate such treatment. I hope that this book will be useful in learning how to make, interpret and take action on such observations.

I should like to thank Michael Buttler, Anne Wade and Peter Tucker of Penguin Education for their considerable help in what otherwise would have been a much more arduous task. I should also like to thank the Coronary Care Unit at Edgware General Hospital for their help in the taking of some of the photographs and to Dr Ted Nathan and Dr Celia Oakley for some of the X-rays used in illustration.

Chapter 1   The circulatory system

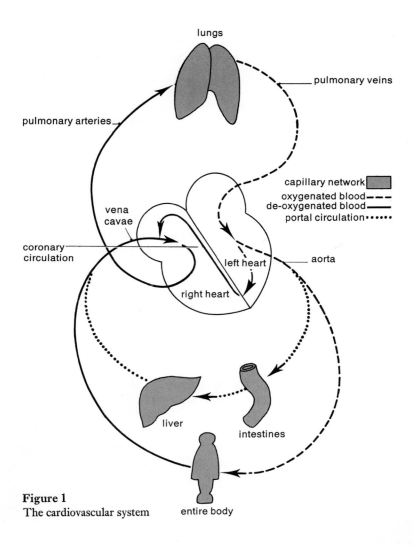

Figure 1
The cardiovascular system

The cardiovascular system (Figure 1) is completely self-contained and consists of the blood vessels, through which the blood circulates, and the heart, which is a pump. There are three parts to the circulatory system: the *systemic system* supplying the body as a whole, the *pulmonary system* supplying the lungs and the *coronary system* supplying the heart muscle itself.

The blood supplies oxygen and other essential nutrients to every cell and tissue in the body, and carries away carbon dioxide and other waste products. Some organs, such as the brain, are so sensitive that they can survive for only a few minutes without the oxygen carried by the blood. Circulation of the blood is essential, for otherwise it would soon be depleted of oxygen and nutrients, and overloaded with waste products.

This circulation takes place through the blood vessels and is pumped by the heart. There are three main types of blood vessel: *arteries, veins* and *capillaries*. The arteries have strong, but elastic, walls and carry the blood which the heart pumps out in spurts. The elastic walls of the arteries expand and contract, evening out the flow and pressure of the blood. The large artery leaving the left side of the heart is the *aorta*; this divides into smaller branches, which themselves divide again and again to form fine arteries, known as *arterioles*. These subsequently divide further into very fine capillaries. The capillaries have very thin walls which cannot withstand high pressures, so the pressure of the blood is reduced in the arterioles, which have thick, muscular but relatively inelastic walls, and a narrow bore.

The capillaries receive blood from the arterioles and pass it into the *venules* which drain into the veins. The veins carry the blood away from the tissues and back to the heart. The pressure in the veins is always low, so they need only thin walls, and they are larger and more commodious than the arteries. Many of the veins, especially in the limbs, have valves which prevent the blood flowing backwards.

The muscles, and hence the bore, of the blood vessels are controlled by the sympathetic (*thoracolumbar*) part of the autonomic nervous system. This enables the amount of blood going to different tissues to be varied. Some limb muscles need very little blood while they are at rest but, in active exercise, they need a great deal.

The circulatory system supplies the various tissues and organs of the body with the nutrients they require and also removes their waste products. This exchange occurs from the smallest blood vessels, the capillaries, where the nutrients in the blood diffuse through the capillary walls into the cells of the body, and the waste products diffuse in the opposite direction, out of the cells and into the capillaries. During its circulation through the lungs, the blood is charged with oxygen, and discharges its carbon dioxide. Other waste products are discharged when the blood passes through the kidneys. Nutrient material is collected during its passage through the gut and the liver. In these ways, the blood maintains a supply of nutrients to all the cells of the body.

The heart

In order to keep the blood moving in the circulatory system, a pump is essential. The heart is this pump. In fact, it is a double pump, its right side serving the lungs and its left side serving the rest of the body.

The heart is a conical, hollow, muscular structure which is situated in the middle of the thorax. It measures about 13 cm from the base (at the top) to the apex (below) and 9 cm at its widest point. It weighs about 300 g in a man and about 225 g in a woman. It is made up of three layers – thin *endocardium* on the inside, thick *myocardium* (muscle) in the middle and thin *pericardium* covering it on the outside.

There are four chambers in the heart (Figure 2), the *left atrium*, the *right atrium*, the *left ventricle* and the *right ventricle*. The left and right sides of the heart are completely separated from base to apex by two septa. The two atrial chambers (the upper chambers) have thin walls and collect the blood from the great veins. The left atrium collects the blood from the *pulmonary veins*, and the right atrium collects the blood from the *superior and inferior vena cavae* (Figure 3). The two ventricles (the lower chambers) have thick walls, the left much thicker than the right. These chambers pump blood. The left ventricle pumps it into the *aorta* through the *aortic valve* and the right into the *pulmonary artery* through the *pulmonary valve*.

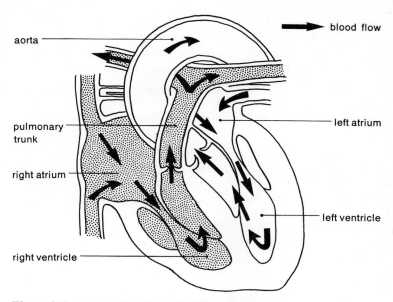

Figure 2 Structure and pumping function of the heart

Each atrium is separated from its corresponding ventricle by a valve. The right atrium and the right ventricle are separated by the *tricuspid valve*. Blood from the inferior and superior vena cava and from the coronary sinus (which drains the heart muscle) enters the right atrium, passing through the tricuspid valve into the right ventricle, which then

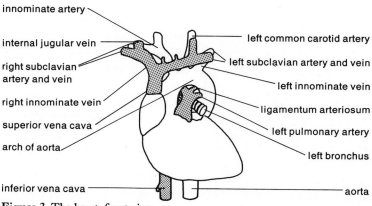

Figure 3 The heart, front view

pumps it through the pulmonary valve into the pulmonary artery. On the left side, the valve is known as the *mitral valve*.

The left atrium receives blood from the four pulmonary veins and passes it through the mitral valve into the left ventricle, which then pumps it through the *aortic valve* into the aorta. The ventricles may be regarded as having an inflow and outflow tract. Inflow is from the atrium to the body of the ventricle and the outflow tract is from the body towards the great arteries.

The heart beats about 70 times per minute. The atria contract first, the right atrium starting slightly before the left, then the ventricles contract, the left ventricle starting slightly before the right. The contraction of the heart is known as *systole*, relaxation as *diastole*. The activation of the

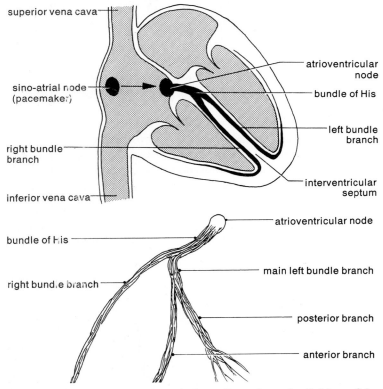

Figure 4 The conduction system; the lower figure shows the divisions of the main left bundle branch

muscles of the heart is carried out by groups of specialized neuromuscular cells known as *the conduction system* (Figure 4). The impulse which begins the electrical activity resulting in the contraction of the heart is normally from the group of cells known as the *sino-atrial node*. This is situated between the right atrium and the superior vena cava and is extremely rhythmic. From here, the impulse passes through the atrium to the *atrioventricular node*, which lies in the floor of the right atrium near the membranous part of the septum which separates the left and right ventricles (the *interventricular septum*). From there, the impulse passes via conducting tissue known as the *bundle of His* situated at the top of the muscular part of the interventricular septum where it divides into the right and left bundle branches. The right branch runs down the right side of the septum giving off smaller branches as it goes, then in a band to the whole of the right ventricle. The left branch passes down the left side of the septum and then divides into two more branches, the anterior and posterior branches. These pass to the base of the corresponding papillary muscles and break up into the *Purkinje* network which supplies the whole of the left ventricle. Thus the rhythmic impulse starting at the sino-atrial node (also known as the *pacemaker*) spreads through both atria to the atrioventricular node, from where it is transmitted into the two ventricles, resulting in the contraction of the heart.

During the *refractory period* after each contraction, any stimulus reaching the muscle cells will be ineffective. One of the ways in which the drug *digoxin* slows the heart is by prolonging the refractory period.

Blood is supplied to the heart by the *coronary arteries*, which are perhaps the most important blood vessels in the body. They begin at the root of the aorta and run into the heart wall, where they form a network of capillaries. Blood is collected from these capillaries into the *coronary veins*, which empty into the coronary sinus and thus into the right atrium.

The development of the heart

During the first two weeks of embryonic life, the heart develops from a straight tube which becomes twisted into an S-shape. Constrictions then divide it into five parts, the *sinus venosus* (into which the veins of the body drain), the *common atrium*, the *common ventricle*, the *bulbus cordis* and the *truncus arteriosus* (see Figure 60). Later in development, the septa appear which divide the atrial and ventricular chambers into the left and right parts. The atria and ventricles are separated by the growth of endocardial cushions which also form the mitral and tricuspid valves. A spiral dividing wall (or septum) is formed in the bulbus cordis and the truncus arteriosus, dividing them into the paths out of the ventricles (outflow tracts) and into the aorta and pulmonary artery. The heart has more or less assumed its adult form by the second month of foetal life.

The foetus obtains its nutrition across the placenta in which the mother's circulation runs close to the foetal circulation (see Figure 61). The blood of the foetus becomes oxygenated in this way. It leaves the placenta in the *umbilical veins* which lead into the *ductus venosus* on the inferior surface of the foetal liver. The ductus venosus is joined by the *portal vein* draining the gut and then runs into the inferior vena cava bringing arterial blood to the right atrium. Only slight mixing occurs here, as most blood is diverted through the *foramen ovale* (a passage between the atria), still open in the foetus, to the left atrium, left ventricle and aorta. The venous blood returning to the right atrium via the superior vena cava flows through the tricuspid valve into the right ventricle and then into the pulmonary artery. However, the foetus is not breathing, so the lungs do not need much blood. Thus the blood is shunted from the pulmonary artery through the *ductus arteriosus* to the descending aorta. This becomes a channel for the venous blood leaving the foetus. It runs into the *umbilical arteries* which arise from the internal iliac arteries of the foetus, and these take the blood back to the placenta, where it is oxygenated again.

When the baby is born, air is breathed into the lungs and more blood flows into them. Also, more blood flows back from the lungs to the left atrium, so the foramen ovale closes. The midwife ties the umbilical cord, and the ductus arteriosus closes. These physiological changes happen very rapidly, but it is several months before the channels are completely obliterated, though the adult pattern of circulation is quickly reached after birth.

Electrophysiology of the heart and electrocardiography

All nurses, especially those in Coronary Care Units, should have some knowledge of electrocardiography. This is a process whereby the electrical changes in the beating heart are recorded on a moving paper chart, and it is an essential part of the examination of the cardiovascular system.

The conduction system of the heart is described on page 14. The impulse which travels from the sino-atrial node to the ventricles resulting in the contraction of the heart is electrical in nature, but the forces are so small that they cannot be detected by a galvanometer. However, these small forces stimulate contractions of the atria and ventricles and the electrical changes of these large masses of muscle are much greater, and can be detected and recorded. The origin of the electricity is in the membrane of the myocardial cells and is caused by the chemical changes that take place there.

The cell membrane can stop sodium ions (Na^+) getting into the inside of the cell, so there are normally more sodium ions outside the cell than in it. This results in the membrane having a positive charge on the outside surface and a negative charge on the inside. The resting cell is said to be *polarized*. When the cell contracts, sodium ions pass into the cell and the electrical state changes. It is then said to be *depolarized*. The cell then returns to its normal resting state in a process of *repolarization*.

These electrical changes are detected by a galvanometer which records a graph on special squared paper. The electrodes of the galvanometer are arranged so that an electric current moving towards the electrode causes the recording pen to deflect upwards, and a current moving away from it causes the pen to deflect downwards. The electrode leads are attached to different places on the patient's limbs and chest. A special conducting jelly (containing salt) is rubbed into the skin, and the electrode is then secured over it with an elastic strap (or a suction cap in the case of the leads on the chest). The paper is divided by thick lines into 5 mm squares and these are subdivided with thinner lines into 1 mm squares. The paper is arranged to move under the galvanometer pen at 25 mm per second, so one large square corresponds to 0·2 seconds. The instrument is standardized so that 1 millivolt causes a pen deflection of 1 cm (2 large squares).

The electrocardiograph leads

There are twelve leads which provide twelve separate traces. These are made up of three *standard leads*, three *unipolar limb leads* and six *chest leads* (Figure 5). Each lead consists of two electrodes: the *exploring electrode*, which is the positive electrode and picks up the electrical impulse from the heart, and the *indifferent electrode*, which is the pathway for the return of the electric current to complete the circuit.

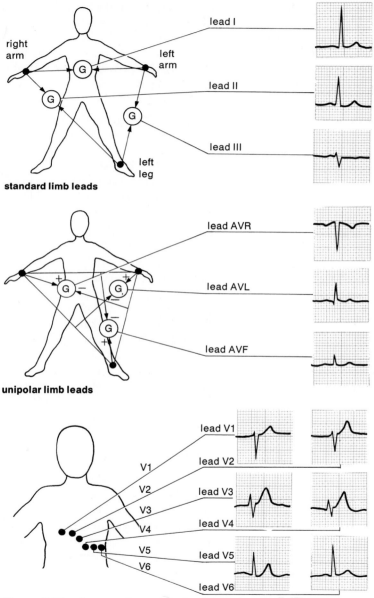

Figure 5 The electrocardiograph leads (G = galvanometer)

The arrangement of the standard leads is as follows:

Lead I The exploring electrode is attached to the left arm and the indifferent electrode to the right arm.

Lead II The exploring electrode is attached to the left leg, and the indifferent electrode to the right arm.

Lead III The exploring electrode is attached to the left leg and the indifferent electrode to the left arm.

The unipolar limb leads are arranged so that the exploring electrode is on one of the limbs and the indifferent electrode is on all the other limbs collectively:

Lead AVR is attached to the right arm.
Lead AVL is attached to the left arm.
Lead AVF is attached to the left leg.

'A' stands for augmented, since the voltages are very low and are increased to make them comparable with those from the other leads. Lead AVR can be regarded as looking at the right side of the heart, lead AVL at the left side, and lead AVF at the inferior surface of the heart. These leads are very useful in clinical diagnosis.

There are six chest leads, labelled V1 to V6, in which the exploring electrode is the one on the chest and the indifferent electrode is connected to all four limbs together. Leads V1 and V2 respectively are placed in the fourth intercostal space on the right and left of the sternum. The fourth intercostal space is found by counting down from the second which lies immediately below the ridge on the upper sternum (angle of Louis). V4 is in the fifth space at the mid-clavicular line. V3 is placed between V2 and V4. V5 and V6 are on a level with V4 at the anterior and mid-axillary lines respectively. The chest leads may be regarded as giving a view of the electrical activity of the heart in the horizontal plane while the standard and unipolar leads give a view in the frontal plane.

The electrocardiogram

The normal trace (Figure 6) takes the form of a series of waves, called the P, Q, R, S and T waves. The appearance of the trace varies from lead to lead. The P wave represents the contraction of the atria, the Q, R and S waves represent the contraction of the ventricles (depolarization) and the T wave represents the relaxation of the ventricles (repolarization). The

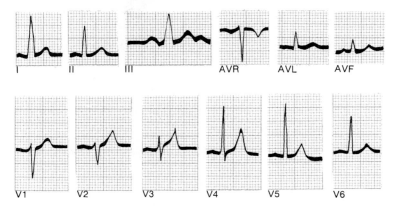

Figure 6 The normal electrocardiogram

repolarization of the atria produces a wave, but it is of such low voltage that it is usually not observed.

The normal electrocardiogram (ECG) is dominated by the left ventricle, which is the greatest mass of muscle in the heart. If an electrode is placed over the left ventricle, the P wave, representing the activity of the atria, will be followed by a Q wave since the first part of the ventricle to be activated is the interventricular septum from the left bundle. This is negative, since the forces are moving away from the electrode.

Then the mass of the ventricle is activated with the electrical forces moving towards the electrode, resulting in a large positive R wave. This pattern is found in leads V5 and V6. But an electrode over the right side of the heart, such as lead VI, produces a different pattern.

It begins with a small R wave as the electrical forces are now moving towards the electrode through the septum. Then, as the right ventricular forces are overcome by the huge left ventricular forces, the R wave is followed by a deep S wave since these forces are moving away from the electrode. These two patterns are the two extremes – the balanced pattern has an equal R and S wave, although the position of this varies from individual to individual, depending on the position of the heart about its vertical axis, usually occurring in V3 or V4.

The position of the heart in the chest will also influence the standard and unipolar limb leads. For example, if the heart is in a horizontal position, the left ventricular pattern would be most marked in lead AVL, whereas if the heart is in the vertical position, it will be most marked in lead AVF. There are infinite variations between these extremes, and the most usual electrocardiogram is produced when the heart is in a position mid-way between them.

The electrocardiogram can give a great deal of information about abnormalities in the rate and rhythm of the heart, and of the pathway taken by the electrical impulses. Hypertrophy of the ventricles may be shown up, as may injury to heart muscle. It is particularly useful in diagnosing ischaemic heart disease (see Chapter 3). The electrocardiogram traces will be discussed in connection with the abnormalities concerned.

Summary of nursing points

The nurse should understand the role of the heart, the blood and the blood vessels in the context of the person's physiology as a whole. She should understand how these organs develop, thus assisting her to understand more clearly any subsequent pathology, particularly if of a congenital nature. She should revise the anatomy of the heart and blood vessels and appreciate events that take place during one heart cycle (physical and electrical); she should also revise the systemic, pulmonary, foetal and portal circulations. The principles of electrophysiology and electrocardiography must be understood, so that later, when these subjects are discussed in more detail in relation to disease, they will be more meaningful.

It would be useful for the nurse to know the important landmarks in history; for example, the discovery of the circulation of the blood in 1628 by William Harvey; this would give her a greater insight into this vital system.

Chapter 2   Heart failure

If nothing can be done or is done about the cause of most kinds of heart disease, heart failure will eventually occur. This does not usually imply the death of the patient, but a condition in which part of the heart is failing. It may be the left, the right or both sides of the heart that are in trouble and need help. Heart failure has been regarded: as an abnormal response to changes in the filling pressure, i.e. on the venous side; as an inability of the heart to empty itself adequately, thus leading to congestion behind it (*backward failure*); or as an inability to maintain adequate circulation to all the tissues of the body (*forward failure*). It is impossible to define heart failure in terms of cardiac output, since this varies so widely from one person to another, and in the same person at different times. Even so, the failing heart will not respond adequately to any additional demands, such as exercise. Effective treatment is perfectly possible and this has been known for many years.

The cardiac cycle

Each contraction and filling of the heart takes about 0·8 seconds (Figure 7). Starting with systole, the ventricles begin to contract. When the pressure in the ventricles is greater than the pressure in the atria, then the mitral and tricuspid valves close, so the blood will not be lost back into the atrial chambers. The ventricles continue to contract and, when the pressure is greater than that in the aorta on the left side and the pulmonary artery on the right side, then the aortic and pulmonary valves open and blood flows into the aorta and the pulmonary artery. Most of the blood in the ventricles will be driven out. When contraction has finished, and systole ended, the pressure in the ventricles begins to fall. When it is below that in the aorta and the pulmonary artery, then the aortic and pulmonary valves close so that blood will not flow back into the heart and be lost to the systemic and pulmonary circulations. The pressure will continue to fall and, when it is nearly zero, the mitral and tricuspid valves will open and the ventricles will begin to fill again.

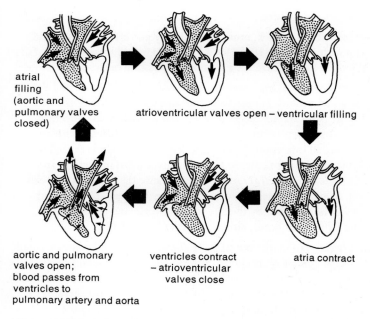

atrial filling (aortic and pulmonary valves closed)

atrioventricular valves open – ventricular filling

aortic and pulmonary valves open; blood passes from ventricles to pulmonary artery and aorta

ventricles contract – atrioventricular valves close

atria contract

Figure 7 The cardiac cycle

The flow of blood from the atria to the ventricles is at first passive, and occupies most of diastole. However, just before the end of diastole, the atria contract, forcefully driving more blood into the now distended ventricles. This is an important contribution to cardiac output. At each systole, the adult heart pumps about 75 ml of blood: this is called the *stroke volume*. If this is multiplied by the heart rate, it will give the *cardiac output*, which is usually about five litres per minute at rest. The heart rate is controlled by the autonomic nervous system, being slowed by the vagus nerve fibres which reach it and increased by the sympathetic nerve fibres. Stroke volume depends on diastolic filling and the venous filling pressure.

Respiration influences the filling of the heart, for in inspiration the negative pressure in the chest is decreased even further and more blood is 'dragged' into the right atrium from the great veins, the superior and inferior vena cavae. Also, because of the increased volume of the lungs in inspiration, blood is held back in them and left-sided filling is diminished. The opposite situation occurs during expiration.

Left ventricular failure

The left ventricle is a thick, muscular and very powerful structure and it puts up with enormous strain for a long time before it fails. It may fail gradually or acutely. There are a number of possible causes.

A coronary thrombosis may present as left-sided heart failure, and the pain may go unnoticed. It may also occur more gradually in ischaemic heart disease (see Chapter 3), with or without angina. Some degree of left ventricular failure occurs in about 75 per cent of patients with an acute myocardial infarction. Sometimes, left-sided failure is caused by an aneurysm of the left ventricle following myocardial infarction, and sometimes it is due to *mitral regurgitation* because the papillary muscles have been damaged by ischaemic heart disease. Untreated high blood pressure will be tolerated by the left ventricle for many years, but eventually failure will occur, either gradually or suddenly.

In mitral regurgitation, the mitral valve allows blood to flow back through it in systole so the left ventricle has to work harder to maintain cardiac output. Because part of its effort is wasted, left-sided failure will eventually occur if the regurgitation is sufficiently severe. Severe aortic stenosis or regurgitation through the aortic valve places a great strain on the left ventricle and, although it will hypertrophy and cope for a little while, it will eventually fail. Also, if the heart muscle is damaged by any process such as a cardiomyopathy, it will eventually fail.

When the left ventricular muscle fails, it is unable to expel all the blood that it contains. Thus, the pressure at the end of diastole fails to fall to zero, and is instead raised, so the pressure needed to fill the ventricle must be increased, and the pressure in the left atrium goes up. Since there are no valves between the left atrium and the pulmonary veins, the pressure in the pulmonary veins also increases. When the pressure becomes sufficiently high, fluid is forced out of the circulation into the alveoli, and *oedema* of the lungs results. Normally, the osmotic pressure of the plasma keeps this fluid in the blood vessels but, at the pressure levels encountered in a failing left ventricle, this is not possible and the patient may literally drown. If there is excess fluid in the alveoli, the blood cannot be oxygenated properly so, to overcome this, the respiratory rate is increased. The fluid also stiffens the lungs and makes the work of breathing more difficult.

Symptoms and signs
One of the most common symptoms in left ventricular failure (Figure 8) is *dyspnoea* (breathlessness) on exertion. It may also be associated with a dry cough. Dyspnoea in heart failure may be divided into four grades:

Grade 1 Mild – occurs only with unusual exertion such as running or walking uphill.

Grade 2 Moderate – occurs walking on the level.

Grade 3 Severe – walking impossible, even slowly on the level.

Grade 4 Gross – so breathless that the patient is practically confined to bed.

Breathlessness on lying flat (*orthopnoea*) may also occur; it is relieved by sitting up. *Paroxysmal nocturnal dyspnoea* is very characteristic of left ventricular failure. The patient is suddenly awakened by severe dyspnoea,

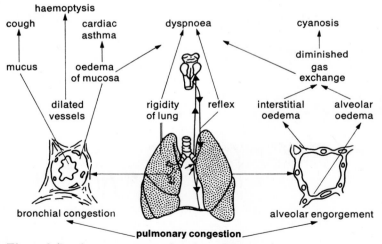

Figure 8 Respiratory symptoms from heart failure

which causes him to sit up or to get up for air. There may be a dry cough and wheezing. The attack gradually passes off. *Acute pulmonary oedema* may occur. There is sudden breathlessness associated with a cough producing copious frothy sputum, which may be tinged pink by blood from the rupture of some pulmonary capillaries by the high intravascular pressure. The patient may be cyanosed and sweating with a rapid pulse and a raised blood pressure.

Because of the excess fluid in the alveoli, moist sounds called *crepitations* may be heard with a stethoscope, particularly in the lower part of the lungs. This is a most valuable physical sign. Pleural effusions, usually small, may also occur because the veins of the visceral pleura drain into the pulmonary veins and are therefore subject to the high pressure of left-sided failure. The heart may be clinically enlarged, with evidence of left ventricular hypertrophy. An abnormal ventricular filling sound, a third heart sound, may be heard.

Chest X-rays may be very characteristic, showing enlarged pulmonary veins, shadows produced by the fluid in the alveoli, and also horizontal lines at the bases of the lungs due to fluid in the walls between the lung lobules.

Left ventricular hypertrophy may show up on the ECG (Figure 9), in which both the QRS complex (representing ventricular depolarization) and the T wave (representing ventricular repolarization) may be affected.

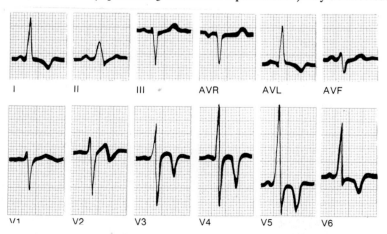

Figure 9 Electrocardiogram of left ventricular hypertrophy

The leads facing the left ventricle (V5 and V6) show increased voltage of the R waves, whereas those opposite (V1 and V2) show abnormally deep S waves. There may be some widening of the QRS complex and, if the interventricular septum is hypertrophied, prominent Q waves may be seen in V5 and V6. As the hypertrophy becomes more severe, the T waves become flattened and eventually inverted in the leads with the tall R waves. The ST segments may be depressed.

Treatment

If the patient is seated upright with his legs down, either on the edge of the bed or on a chair, this should result in a rapid fall in the pressure in the pulmonary veins, and the symptoms will be relieved. Tourniquets are easily applied to the limbs and lead to a fall in pressure because of decreased venous return to the heart. Oxygen through a face mask is helpful and is also of psychological benefit to the patient: it can easily be given by the nurse. However, drugs are often needed, and heroin (5 mg) or morphine (10 mg) given intravenously (provided there is no chronic lung disease with respiratory failure) may bring dramatic relief.

Aminophylline (500 mg given slowly intravenously) may also give relief and help bronchospasm. If there is any doubt whether the 'asthma' is cardiac or respiratory, aminophylline is the drug to use. Frusemide (20 to 40 mg given intravenously) initiates a rapid diuresis (flow of urine) and relief of the pulmonary oedema and symptoms. If the patient has not been taking digoxin, an intravenous dose of 0·5–1·0 mg may be given, and the drug then continued by mouth. If the treatment is not rapidly effective, intermittent positive-pressure respiration with a ventilator may save life. If this has to be continued for many days, a tracheostomy (surgical intubation of the trachea) will be necessary.

Right ventricular failure

The right ventricle is not nearly so sturdy a structure as the left, and fails more readily. There are, again, several possible causes. It may be secondary to left ventricular failure.

If chronic left-sided failure persists, the raised pressure in the venous capillaries necessitates a rise in the pressure in the arterial capillaries in order to maintain the forward flow of blood. This means in turn that the pressures in the pulmonary artery and the right ventricle have to be increased. The right ventricle *hypertrophies* (enlarges) to provide power for the higher pressures, and may maintain them for many years, but will eventually fail. Thus, the end result of any of the causes given above for left ventricular failure will eventually be right-sided failure (*congestive cardiac failure*) as well.

Right ventricular failure due to an increase in pressure in the pulmonary arteries may also arise in other ways. There may be disease of the lungs, such as chronic bronchitis and emphysema. There may also be obstruction to the pulmonary arterioles, such as when numerous emboli (clots) from a thrombus (clot formed on the lining of a blood vessel) in the legs or pelvic veins lodge in the lungs.

In *mitral stenosis*, because of the obstruction at the valve, the pressure rises in the left atrium and, therefore, also in the pulmonary veins. This necessitates a rise in pressure in the pulmonary arterioles to maintain forward flow, and the arterioles tend to thicken, creating resistance to the flow. This causes considerable increases of pressure in the main pulmonary arteries and the right ventricle. In all these situations, the right ventricle will eventually fail.

In the congenital abnormality, *atrial septal defect*, the right side of the heart may be handling much more blood than it usually does. In middle or later adult life, if the defect has not been closed surgically, the right side of the heart may fail, particularly if there is also atrial fibrillation which is common.

If the tricuspid valve allows regurgitation of blood into the right atrium, the right ventricle will eventually fail. If the tricuspid valve is stenosed, there will be an increase of venous pressure and a picture similar to that of congestive cardiac failure, although the right ventricle has not failed. The ring surrounding the tricuspid valve is not a very strong structure, and in congestive heart failure it commonly stretches, so that the tricuspid valve allows regurgitation into the right atrium. This is often called *functional tricuspid regurgitation*, to distinguish it from that due to a diseased tricuspid valve. It often disappears on treatment. In severe narrowing of the pulmonary valve, usually a congenital abnormality, the strain on the right ventricle is enormous. It will hypertrophy and deal with the high pressure involved for many years but, unless corrected surgically, it will eventually fail.

The mechanism of right ventricular failure is complex. If the right ventricle cannot pump enough blood forward to match the venous blood flowing into it, the venous pressure in the systemic circulation rises.

This leads to distension of the veins, distension of the liver, and to oedema. The oedema arises because the osmotic pressure keeping the fluid in the peripheral venous capillaries is overcome by the hydrostatic pressure within the capillaries. The cardiac output is inadequate, so the blood supply to various organs is redistributed. The kidneys are affected more than any other organs, which results in increased retention of sodium in the body and therefore an increase in the amount of fluid in the body. This makes the oedema worse.

Symptoms and signs
The most important sign of right-sided heart failure (Figure 10) is raised pressure in the jugular veins (Figure 11). The patient should be propped up in bed on pillows at an angle of about 45 degrees. Look at the internal jugular vein (ignore the external jugular veins) in the anterior triangle of the neck in front of the sternomastoid muscle. It may be distinguished from the carotid artery by the fact that light pressure with the finger, below the gently pulsating upper level of the blood column, will stop the

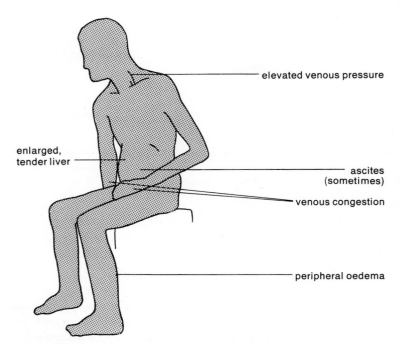

Figure 10 The effects of right ventricular failure

pulsation. In addition, pressure on the abdomen, particularly over the liver, will send the level up. It is often useful to measure and chart the pressure in this vein. In a normal individual, the pressure does not exceed 2 cm above the *sternal angle*, the protuberance which can be felt over the upper sternum just above the second intercostal space (Figure 11).

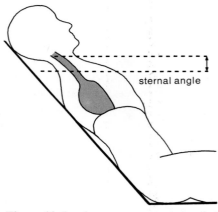

Figure 11 Jugular venous pressure; vertical height above the sternal angle represents the pressure in the right atrium

Another important sign is oedema. The patient will often complain of swelling of the ankles, which usually worsens as the day goes on and disappears after a night in bed.

A patient already in bed will have most of the oedema in the sacral and lumbar regions, and the feet may show nothing at all. A characteristic of cardiac oedema is that it pits on pressure. As the heart failure worsens, the extent of the oedema increases, until it reaches even the arms, chest wall and face. Occasionally, pleural effusions and *ascites* (accumulation of fluid in the peritoneum) may also occur. The liver may be felt to be enlarged in the abdomen, and is usually tender due to distension of the capsule, unless the failure is of long standing.

The heart may be clinically enlarged and there may be evidence of left and right ventricular hypertrophy. An abnormal ventricular filling sound (third heart sound) may be heard. The long systolic murmur of functional tricuspid valve regurgitation may also be heard. The patient may also be dyspnoeic because of left-sided failure, and general fatigue is a common complaint. Nausea and vomiting may occur owing to the distension of

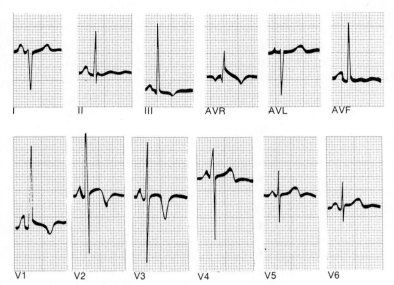

Figure 12 Electrocardiogram of right ventricular hypertrophy

veins in the stomach. Abdominal pain because of distension of the liver may be the chief complaint. Mild jaundice may occur and in the very late stages there may be considerable loss of body tissue (*cardiac cachexia*).

Right ventricular hypertrophy may be shown up on the ECG (Figure 12). The leads facing the right ventricle (V1 and AVR) show dominant R waves instead of the normal S. There may also be inversion of the T waves in the right chest leads and deep S waves over the left chest leads. There is commonly right atrial hypertrophy as well.

Treatment
It is usually necessary to treat the failure itself first but, once the situation is controlled, it is possible to consider whether the cause of the failure can be remedied. For example, should a faulty valve be replaced, or should a congenital abnormality be corrected surgically? Bed rest is very useful, particularly in the earlier stages of treatment. Heart work is reduced, venous pressure falls and a diuresis may occur spontaneously. Rapid improvement often occurs with bed rest alone.

However, bed rest must not be too prolonged, for it also encourages the development of venous thrombosis and resultant pulmonary embolism.

Mental rest is also important, and the judicious use of sedatives such as diazepam (Valium) in 2–5 mg doses three times a day may be helpful. Oxygen may sometimes be needed, and is given by mask. It often makes the patient feel more secure. Only rarely is ventilation through a tracheostomy tube needed.

Small light meals are usually all that the patient desires. Sometimes, it may help to stop all added salt or to replace it with a proprietary potassium salt instead of the usual sodium one, but only rarely (e.g. in intractable failure) does it become necessary to restrict sodium.

Digoxin is the usual preparation of digitalis used, and is the most valuable drug in the treatment of most patients with heart failure. It increases the strength of myocardial contraction, both in the normal and the failing heart, and it also slows the rate of the heart, thus allowing adequate filling time before systole. It does this by vagal stimulation and by depressing conduction from the atria to the ventricles, prolonging the refractory period of the atrioventricular node (see p. 15). It leads to a diuresis because of the improved cardiac output and increased renal blood flow.

Digoxin is excreted in the urine, and the object of treatment is to build up the concentration in heart muscle until maximum benefit is obtained, and then to replace the daily loss in the urine. The dose required varies greatly from patient to patient, and the line between toxic and therapeutic doses is very narrow, so that great care is needed. Treatment by mouth is usually sufficient, so 0·5–1·0 mg may be given at once, followed by 0·25 mg six-hourly for two or three days, after which once or twice a day is usually sufficient. As people become older and renal function diminishes, much smaller doses may be needed – even as little as 0·0625 mg ($\frac{1}{4}$ tablet) being all that is required. Special P G (paediatric geriatric) tablets are available. If very rapid digitalization is needed, then 0·5–1·0 mg may be given intramuscularly or intravenously. The intravenous route is potentially dangerous, as *ventricular fibrillation* (rapid uncoordinated twitching of the ventricular muscle fibres) may result.

Although it is very useful, digoxin has marked toxic effects which must be watched for carefully. The nurse is often the first to notice these and must bring them to the attention of the doctor. The early effects are general malaise, headache, nausea, anorexia (loss of appetite) and vomiting. There may be abdominal pain and diarrhoea. Usually, if the drug is stopped for a day or two and then resumed in a smaller dose, these will disappear. Much more serious are the disturbances in heart rhythm, which not infrequently occur without any prior complaint of nausea. The most common is ventricular ectopic beats, often occurring every second beat leading to 'coupling'. This is a signal to reduce the dose. Other common abnormal rhythms are atrial *tachycardia* (unduly rapid beat), often with block, usually two to one, ventricular tachycardia and fibrillation, and any degree of heart block. If any of these occur or if the pulse rate becomes very slow the doctor should be informed immediately. If a rapid regular rate is observed, it may be an atrial tachycardia and, if digoxin is continued or increased in dosage, death may occur. Digoxin toxicity is worse if potassium stores in the body are low. Since this tends to occur with many diuretics, it is most important that potassium supplements are taken as prescribed.

Other preparations of digitalis are *digitoxin*, which is excreted more slowly than digoxin, and *lanatoside C*, which is a little more rapid in action.

If digoxin on its own is not sufficient, other diuretics will be needed. *Thiazides* are commonly used and seem to work by inhibiting the reabsorption of sodium in the distal tubule of the kidney. Some of the commonly used ones are cyclopenthiazide (Navidrex) 0·5–1·0 mg daily, bendroflumethiazide (Neonaclex) 5 mg daily and chlorothiazide (Saluric) 0·5–1·0 g daily. These drugs tend to lead to potassium depletion, so it is important to give the patient potassium supplements such as slow–release tablets (Slow 'K') 600 mg two or three times a day. Potassium tablets occasionally lead to ulceration, bleeding or even *stenosis* (narrowing) of the small bowel. Some toxic effects of thiazides are diabetes, gout, skin rashes (occasionally) and (rarely) serious blood diseases. Another very powerful diuretic is *frusemide* (Lasix). This has a rapid action, which means that if taken early in the day the inconvenience of the diuresis is over in a few hours. It prevents the reabsorption of sodium and also leads to considerable potassium loss, so potassium supplements are essential. It is usually taken by mouth in doses of from 40–120 mg daily, although it may be used intravenously in doses of 20–40 mg. This can be very useful in acute left ventricular failure. Ethacrynic acid (Edecrin), 50 mg three times a day, is less often used, but is very powerful. Potassium supplements are also needed with this drug.

Aldosterone is a hormone secreted by the adrenal cortex which causes retention of sodium and loss of potassium by its action on the distal tubule. In some patients with oedema, aldosterone is secreted in excess, making matters worse. The drug *spironolactone* (Aldactone A) prevents this action on the distal tubule, and may lead to a diuresis as a result. It can be very useful, but its action takes several days to become apparent. It also has the advantage that it conserves potassium and may usefully be used, together with one of the other diuretics already discussed. The dosage is 25–50 mg four times a day. *Triamterene* (Dytac) is also useful because it does not lead to potassium depletion. It is used in a dose of 50 mg three times a day.

Intractable heart failure

Usually, with a combination of the drugs discussed, heart failure responds rapidly and satisfactorily, but occasionally this is not so. If the patient is uncomfortable, it may be necessary to remove, mechanically, fluid from the pleural cavity or from the abdomen. Very rarely, fluid may have to be drained from the legs by putting cannulae (Southey's tubes) into the subcutaneous tissues of the *dependent* (hanging down) legs. This should

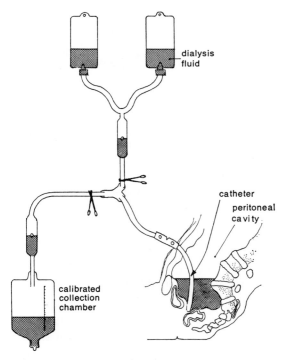

Figure 13 Peritoneal dialysis

be avoided if possible, but a lot of fluid may be removed and a diuresis may follow. In some patients, excess fluid has been removed by peritoneal dialysis (Figure 13).

Maintenance therapy

After a first episode of even severe congestive heart failure, most patients recover, and lead perfectly comfortable lives for many years on maintenance treatment. If a remediable cause of the failure is found, such as thyrotoxicosis, hypertension or an operable mechanical abnormality, then treatment of this may make maintenance treatment unnecessary. In some circumstances, the cause of the failure may improve sufficiently to remove the need for continued treatment. This is commonly the case in the left ventricular failure, frequently seen after a myocardial infarction.

Summary of nursing points

The patient in heart failure may be extremely ill. The nurse must appreciate the main causes, types, clinical signs, investigations and treatment of heart failure.

The care of such a patient makes great demands on the nurse. Constant observation must be maintained of the pulse, blood pressure, colour, character of breathing, and nervous and emotional state, together with the level of morale; this is vital in detecting signs of deterioration in the patient's condition, and ensuring his comfort, correct treatment and recovery.

Accurate observations and records of the patient's general condition, fluid balance, temperature, pulse, respiration and blood pressure must be kept. Should the patient go into cardiac arrest, the nurse must be proficient in carrying out emergency treatment.

Chapter 3   Ischaemic heart disease

The coronary arteries supply the heart muscle with oxygen and nutrients, enabling it to contract and pump blood round the circulatory system. They are the most important arteries in the body, but are also the most likely to become blocked by disease. Disease of the coronary arteries is the most common cause of death in the Western world.

Anatomy of the coronary arteries

There are two coronary arteries, the right and the left (Figure 14). They begin at the root of the aorta, the great blood vessel which leaves the left ventricle. At the aortic root, there are three swellings called the *sinuses*

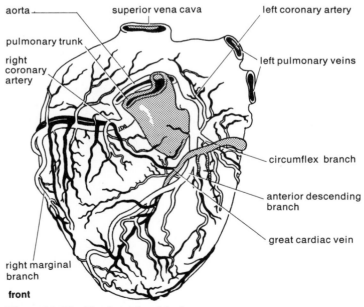

Figure 14 The blood supply of the heart

of Valsalva, which lie above the three cusps of the aortic valve. The coronary arteries begin from two of these sinuses. The *left coronary artery* soon divides into two branches: one, the *anterior descending*, travels down over the anterior wall of the heart, giving off branches to the ventricles and to the septum between them; the other, the *circumflex branch*, swings round the base of the left atrium to reach the inferior or diaphragmatic surface of the heart, giving off branches to the left atrium and to the left ventricle, and finally *anastomosing* (mingling) with the terminal branches of the right coronary artery. The *right coronary artery* sweeps round the base of the right atrium to reach the posterior surface

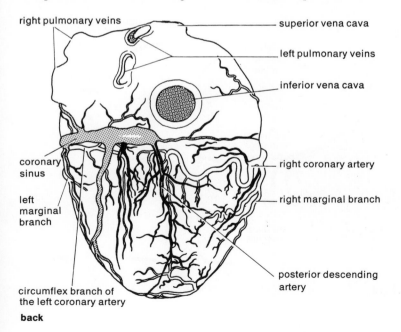

right pulmonary veins

superior vena cava

left pulmonary veins

inferior vena cava

coronary sinus

right coronary artery

left marginal branch

right marginal branch

circumflex branch of the left coronary artery

posterior descending artery

back

of the heart, giving off branches to supply the right atrium, the interventricular septum and both ventricles. In most people, the right coronary artery also gives branches to the sino–atrial node and the conducting system of the heart, although in a few these may come from the left coronary artery. Although individual variations occur, usually the left coronary artery supplies most of the *myocardium* (heart muscle).

The coronary circulation

The blood from the coronary arteries passes into an extensive web of small vascular channels coursing among the muscle fibres of the heart, most of it is then returned to the coronary veins, which run parallel to the branches of the coronary arteries. These terminate in the coronary sinus on the inferior surface of the heart, and discharge black, exhausted blood into the right atrium. Some blood perfuses through the myocardium directly into the heart chambers. In most arteries, forward flow is greatest when the ventricles contract but, because of the great pressure exerted on the wall of the coronary arteries by the contracting ventricle, little flow occurs during *systole* (phase of contraction), most

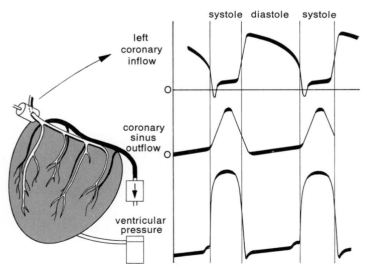

Figure 15 Coronary flow during the cardiac cycle

occurring during *diastole* (phase of relaxation). This is more marked in the left ventricle, which is larger and more powerful than the right (Figure 15). The myocardium removes much more oxygen from the blood flowing through it than do other tissues; hence the black colour of the deoxygenated blood entering the right atrium from the coronary sinus.

The extra oxygen required by the heart when it is working harder, for example in running, can only be obtained by increasing the flow of blood through the coronary vessels. These arteries increase in size if there is lack of oxygen in the blood. This appears to be the most important means of regulating coronary blood flow and increasing the oxygen supply to the heart muscle, enabling it to work harder and increase its output.

Atheroma of the coronary arteries

Disease of the coronary arteries causes them to narrow (Figure 16) or close completely. This reduces or cuts off the blood supply to a part of the heart muscle and leads to *ischaemic heart disease*. From a very early age, changes occur in the walls of the coronary arteries. Fats of varying kinds become incorporated in the walls, which causes fibrous tissue to be formed. This is called *atheroma*, and may obtrude on the *lumen* (inside) of the vessel, or ulcerate into it. On this damaged surface, *thrombosis* (clotting of blood) may cause partial or total blockage, as may also haemorrhage into the atheromatous plaques. Atheroma tends to increase with advancing age, so ischaemic heart disease is more common in the middle and older age groups.

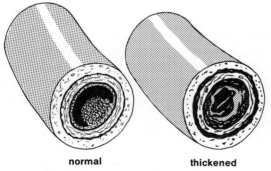

normal   **thickened**

Figure 16 Thickening of the artery walls

The exact cause of the atheroma that leads to ischaemic heart disease is unknown, and several different factors seem to be involved. The disease is more common in men than in women, until the menopause, after which the incidence is the same in both sexes. It certainly tends to run in families. It is more common in those with hypertension, diabetes, myxoedema and gout, and has been shown to be more common in cigarette smokers, in those who live in areas with soft water supplies and in those whose occupations do not require much physical effort. If the cholesterol level in the blood is high, the risk of this disease is increased.

Cholesterol is related to fat metabolism and particularly to fats derived from animals, so dietary causes have been suggested and there is now some evidence to support this. Stress may play a part, but the evidence is not conclusive. However, environmental factors are clearly important. Recently, sugar in the diet has been implicated, but not substantiated.

There are differences in the incidence in different races. The disease is almost unknown in tropical Africa except in the non-indigenous races, yet the incidence in the American Negro has risen steadily over the years until, in some parts of the United States, it now equals the high incidence in the white American. An important study has been going on in America for the last eighteen years, known as the *Framingham study*. In this, 6000 apparently healthy people are being carefully studied. Framingham has found that, of the subjects with a raised cholesterol level, a high blood pressure and evidence (given by an electrocardiograph – see p. 26) of a large left ventricle, 50 per cent developed coronary artery disease within six years.

They found that a man prone to this disease is typically past the age of forty, not very tall, has a cholesterol level in the upper range of normal or above, is somewhat hyperuricaemic or suffering from gout, either himself a diabetic or belonging to a family with a history of diabetes, moderately hypertensive, is a smoker with a quick temper, a hearty eater who does not take much exercise and is therefore to some extent, obese.

The number of cases of coronary thrombosis, particularly in the younger age groups, appears to be increasing. This is not entirely explained by changes in description of causes of death, or by the increase in the population of older people. In England and Wales in 1967, 33 per cent of deaths in men aged 55 to 64 years were attributed to 'arteriosclerotic heart disease' and, in women of similar age, 15 per cent. This number is steadily increasing.

The clinical picture presented by the complete or partial occlusion of the coronary arteries may be of three types: *angina pectoris*, *acute coronary insufficiency* or *myocardial infarction*.

Angina pectoris

This is a pain in the chest caused when the heart muscle does not receive enough blood. It is relieved by rest, and worsened by effort.

The patient is more often a man than a woman, and is usually in middle or later life. The pain is felt in the centre of the chest (Figure 17), often deep to the sternum. It is not felt over the heart or under the left breast. Sometimes it may radiate across or around the chest to one or both shoulders, to one or both arms, even extending to the fingers and thumbs. It may also radiate to the sides of neck and jaws and even to the face and nose. Occasionally, it may begin at the periphery and may never reach the chest at all.

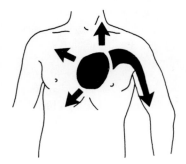

Figure 17 Distribution of anginal pain

The pain is usually described as constricting, crushing or vice-like rather than sharp or stabbing. The patient may sometimes clench his fists against his sternum (Figure 18) and this is often a valuable clue in diagnosis. The pain waxes, becomes constant and then wanes, often lasting no more than a few minutes. It is usually related to exertion and, if the patient stops, the pain disappears. It may be worse after a meal and may be provoked by fear, anger or excitement. Cold weather may also worsen it. Patients whose occupation demands heavy physical exertion may find that they can do their work without trouble, but will experience angina on a slight slope on the way home, or only early in the morning. Angina may be brought on by an unusual posture.

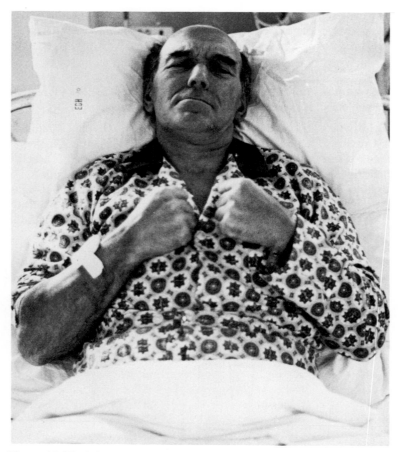

Figure 18 The 'clenched fist' sign of angina

The diagnosis of the condition depends on the doctor taking an accurate history. The pain may be confused with chest pain due to anxiety, or that due to a diaphragmatic hernia. The electrocardiogram may be useful, but is often quite normal.

If the patient is exercised before the electrocardiogram, some abnormalities may show up, but these are difficult to interpret. A recent helpful technique is to stimulate the heart electrically, causing it to beat faster and do more work. The patient with true angina experiences pain at a particular heart rate. This technique can also be used to evaluate the drugs used in treating the condition.

In most cases of angina pectoris, a major coronary artery will eventually be occluded, and lead to *myocardial infarction* (see p. 46). Even so, the average life expectancy from the onset is nine to ten years and about 10 per cent live for as long as twenty years. Women have a better prognosis than men.

Medical treatment

Many patients are only mildly incapacitated, and can lead reasonably normal lives if they understand and are reassured about their symptoms. Obesity should be corrected, and smoking stopped or much reduced, although too much interference in the ways of the really elderly is not justified for it may easily remove their only sources of pleasure. Any underlying condition such as hypertension, anaemia or diabetes is treated. Exercise is helpful, and gradually increasing walking day by day may prove beneficial, although sudden severe exertion should be avoided.

The most useful drug is *glyceryl trinitrate* (trinitrin or TNT). Although it may help relieve prolonged pain, its proper use is as a prophylactic. The usual dose is 0·5 mg, and the tablet should be dissolved under the tongue, or chewed and dissolved in the mouth. It must not be swallowed, for then it is ineffective. Absorption begins rapidly, and the benefit lasts for about thirty minutes. The patient should be instructed to take one a few minutes before commencing any exertion that he knows will cause him pain, and should take as many as he needs. Unpleasant side-effects such as headache and throbbing in the head can usually be overcome by breaking up the tablets to reduce the dose. The patient will learn by experience how much to take to prevent the angina without causing any side-effects. The action of this drug on the heart is not fully understood, but it seems to reduce cardiac work and increase coronary blood flow by widespread *vasodilatation* (widening the blood vessels). The blood pressure may or may not be lowered.

Other, widely used, longer-acting, coronary vasodilator drugs are Sustac, Peritrate, Mycardol, Persantin and Vascardin, but there is no evidence that they are of any value. Similarly, long-term anticoagulant treatment has not been proven useful, in spite of the claims made for it.

The biggest recent advance in the drug treatment of angina has been the advent of drugs known as *beta-blocking drugs*. These block the beta receptors in the sympathetic nervous system so that they are not

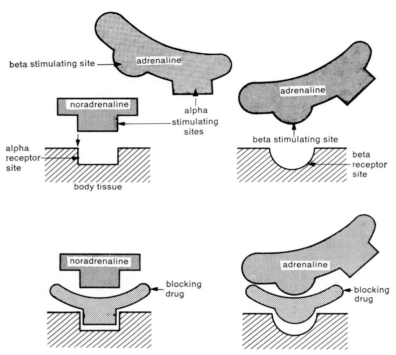

Figure 19 Alpha and beta blocking drugs.
Adrenaline and noradrenaline stimulate certain sites in the body tissue. These are known as alpha and beta receptor sites; alpha receptor stimulation affects the skin, mucous membranes and viscera such as the kidney, while beta receptors influence the heart and bronchial wall muscles. The blocking drugs minimize the action of adrenaline and noradrenaline by preferentially occupying the receptor sites. Beta blocking drugs combat the action of these hormones in the heart

stimulated by adrenalin and noradrenalin (Figure 19). There are many of these receptors in the heart and peripheral blood vessels. One of these drugs is *propanolol* (Inderal), which slows the heart rate and reduces cardiac work. It can greatly reduce the number and severity of the attacks and allow a previously incapacitated patient to lead a normal life again. It is usually started in small doses 10 mg four times a day by mouth and gradually increased to 120 mg four times a day or even more until maximum benefit is obtained. Usually large doses are required. A watch must be kept on the pulse rate and the blood pressure, for both tend to fall and the treatment may have to be abandoned. Heart failure may be precipitated. This may respond to treatment, or the drug may have to be stopped. The drug also affects the sympathetic receptors in the bronchi and may lead to bronchospasm (*asthma*). Recently, other beta-blockers have been used. *Oxyprenolol* (Trasicor), has fewer side-effects but it is not certain that it is as useful as propranolol. More recently cardio-selective drugs, such as Metoprolol (Betaloc and Lopressor) have been introduced.

Surgical treatment
Most patients are sufficiently helped with glyceryl trinitrate, a few need the addition of a beta-blocker. A very small fraction do not get sufficient relief from drugs and, for these, surgery is considered. First, it is necessary to see if the narrowings in the arteries can be treated. The technique is known as *coronary angiography*, and involves passing a special catheter through the brachial artery into the aorta and directly into the openings of the coronary arteries. Radio-opaque dye is injected and excellent pictures of the whole coronary arterial circulation obtained on cine-film.

The most promising operation involves bypassing the areas of narrowing or block with grafts from the patient's own saphenous vein. This technique allows several bad areas to be bypassed. Other, less successful, operations are *direct disobliteration*, in which the atheroma is removed either with instruments or with carbon dioxide under pressure. The results of this operation are disappointing, and the mortality is high. Another operation whose value is uncertain involves the implantation of the internal mammary arteries into the myocardium of the left ventricle. New blood vessels grow and blood flows to the myocardium. The death rate from this operation is very low. It may be more effective to implant the internal mammary artery into the coronary artery beyond the block.

Acute coronary insufficiency

Patients whose suffering is worse than angina, but who have not had a myocardial infarction (although this may be threatened), are said to have acute coronary insufficiency. The pain is anginal pain, coming on suddenly, and often caused by only slight exertion. It may occur even at rest, particularly on lying down.

Some patients who already have angina find it is suddenly much worse. Many patients with myocardial infarction have suffered from angina for

some days beforehand, so acute coronary insufficiency is usually treated
with the hope of preventing myocardial infarction. They should be treated
by bed rest and intravenous *heparin*, followed by *warfarin* by mouth.
Heparin and bed rest should be continued for seven days after the last
bout of chest pain. There is often a dramatic response. Then warfarin can
be given, and the patient is gradually allowed to get up. Warfarin should
be continued for some months. There is now evidence that beta-blocking
drugs may be more effective than anti-coagulants.

Myocardial infarction

Patients suffering from myocardial infarction may have had angina or
even a previous infarction. However, they may have had only vague
symptoms for the previous few days or no warning at all.

The pain resembles that felt in angina, but is more severe and prolonged.
The onset is sudden and usually comes on at rest, but may occur at a
time of emotional crisis or after severe exertion. The pain may last for
half an hour or for several days or until a powerful analgesic is given. The
patient may lose consciousness and have no memory of chest pain.
Occasionally, myocardial infarction may present as an abnormal heart
rhythm with no pain, or as left ventricular failure. Unfortunately,
myocardial infarction often presents as sudden death.

The patient may appear shocked, or perfectly well. He may have a low
blood pressure, an abnormal rhythm or a *tachycardia* (increased heart
rate) and the pulses may sometimes be imperceptible. The pressure in the
jugular veins is often raised in the early stages. An atrial sound is usually
heard, and sometimes a third heart sound. The murmur of mitral
regurgitation is sometimes heard now or later in the illness. The abnormal
systolic outward pulsation of the damaged heart muscle may be felt inside
the apex beat. Crepitations from left ventricular failure may be heard
at the bases of the lungs.

The patient usually runs a fever, with his temperature rising up to
38·5 °C, sometimes for as long as two weeks. The ESR (blood
sedimentation rate) and the white blood count may also be raised. The
electrocardiogram may be normal and even remain normal, but in most
patients there will be a typical pattern in a series of records. It may be
helpful to estimate certain enzymes which are increased and come from the
dead myocardium. Although many tests are used, there are none which are
completely specific for heart muscle. If there is no skeletal disease, such
as a dystrophy, then the CPK (creatine phosphokinase) is the most

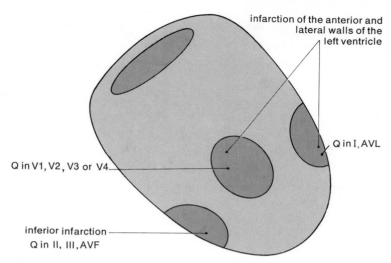

infarction of the anterior and
lateral walls of the
left ventricle

Q in I, AVL

Q in V1, V2, V3 or V4

inferior infarction
Q in II, III, AVF

Figure 20 Sites of myocardial infarction

specific test. A good combination of tests is the SGOT (serum glutamic oxalo-acetic transaminase) test and the LDH (serum lactic dehydrogenase) tests. The SGOT and CPK levels are raised early on, and the LDH is raised after a day or so and lasting a week or even more.

The electrocardiogram will usually show a typical pattern if a series of recordings are made. The changes may be gross or minimal, and reflect the extent of the muscle damage and whether or not the complete thickness of the muscle wall is involved. The most important feature is an abnormal, deep, wide Q wave (because the only electrical impulses are moving away from the electrode). The pattern is usually characteristic with a raised, upwardly convex ST segment and an inverted symmetrical T wave following this. The position and the extent of the infarct (Figure 20) may also be indicated by the electrocardiogram (Figure 21):

1 Extensive *anterior infarction* (Figure 21a) occurring when the left coronary artery is occluded. The pattern is seen in leads I, II, AVL and V1 to V6.

2 *Anteroseptal infarction* (Figure 21b) due to the occlusion of the anterior descending branch of the left coronary artery. The pattern is seen in leads I, AVL and V2 to V4.

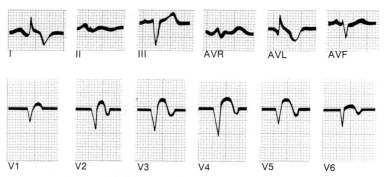

(a) acute extensive anterior myocardial infarction

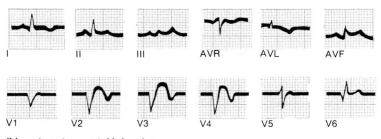

(b) acute anteroseptal infarction

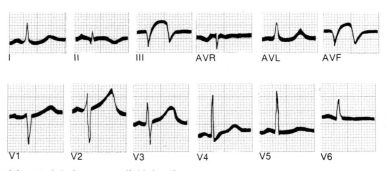

(c) acute inferior myocardial infarction

Figure 21 Electrocardiograms of myocardial infarction

3 *Anterolateral infarction* due to occlusion of the circumflex branch of the left coronary artery. The pattern is seen in leads 1, AVL and V4 to V6.

4 *Inferior infarction* (Figure 21c); here the damaged muscle is on the inferior surface of the left ventricle which lies on the diaphragm. It occurs when the right coronary artery is occluded. It may sometimes extend to involve the posterior wall of the heart and, in some rare cases, infarction of the posterior wall of the heart may occur on its own. The pattern is seen in lead AVF (because it faces the inferior surface of the heart) and also in leads II and III.

As healing takes place, the raised ST segment disappears and the T waves become more deeply inverted. Only occasionally does the electrocardiogram become completely normal.

Complications
Possible complications are abnormal rhythms and shock (see p. 63). Left-sided failure (see p. 24) is common, but congestive failure (see p. 27) is not. Pulmonary embolism (see p. 148) may also occur, as may systemic arterial embolism (see p. 185).

Apart from these, the papillary muscles may be involved in the infarction and lead to mitral regurgitation, usually of mild degree. If severe, the left atrial and pulmonary venous pressures will be very high and pulmonary oedema and severe breathlessness will occur. There will be a loud systolic murmur and a third heart sound. Many patients die but some can be controlled, and the mitral valve replaced surgically. About 10 per cent of deaths are due to rupture of the heart. If this is in the septum a ventricular septal defect (see p. 127) results, usually with severe congestive failure as well. Again, many die but, if the failure can be controlled, surgical repair is possible. If the rupture is of the wall of the heart, death is usually rapid.

After a few days *pericarditis* (inflammation of the pericardium, see p. 158) may occur. If it does, anticoagulants should be stopped because of the risk of haemorrhage into the pericardial sac and *tamponade* (see p. 160). A few patients develop pericarditis much later. This is thought to be an immune reaction from hypersensitivity to dead heart muscle.

An important late complication is a *ventricular aneurysm* (Figure 22a). This is common and usually does not affect the patient's recovery. An aneurysm may even calcify and still give no trouble. But, if it leads to intractable heart failure it can be removed surgically (Figure 22b), often with excellent results.

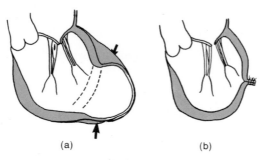

(a)   (b)

Figure 22 Left ventricular aneurysm.
(a) Shows the thin fibrotic aneurysmal left ventricular wall.
(b) The aneurysm is excised to within 1 cm of the viable muscle and the fibrotic
margins are approximated with interrupted sutures

Treatment

Sixty per cent of all patients suffering from myocardial infarction die
before they get to hospital, most of them at home. In hospital, the
existence of special units has reduced the death rate there from this
disease from around 30 per cent to about 15 per cent. The ideal
arrangement is probably to have specially equipped mobile units which
can go immediately to the patient wherever he is. In hospital, it has been
found that the patient is safer in a special Coronary Care Unit than in a
general ward. The Coronary Care Unit is discussed on page 53.

In treatment, relief of pain is the first essential. It is usually necessary to
use an opiate analgesic, preferably *diamorphine hydrochloride* (heroin). The
usual dose is 5 mg, which may be given intramuscularly. If the patient is
shocked, as is often the case, tissue perfusion will be poor, and the
intravenous route should be used. Morphine (15 mg) may also be used
but, since it may lead to hypotension and *bradycardia* (slow heart rate),
nausea and vomiting, it should be combined with *atropine* (0·6 mg).
Perphenazine (Fentazin), 5 mg intramuscularly or by mouth several times
a day, may also control nausea or vomiting. Not every patient needs a
narcotic drug, and some may need no analgesic at all.

An intravenous line should be set up as soon as the patient is admitted
to hospital in order to avoid any delay in administering those drugs which
either have to be, or are more effective when, administered
intravenously. A simple needle technique can be used, or a Teflon or
similar catheter can be passed into the superior vena cava or right atrium.

The same line can also be used when necessary for continuous recording of the right atrial pressure. In order to avoid blood clotting in the needle and tubing, 500 units of heparin are added to 500 ml of 5 per cent dextrose or laevulose which runs in over each twelve-hour period. Automatic drip regulators allow the drip to be easily controlled. Fifty milligrams of hydrocortisone are also added to suppress inflammation at the needle entry site and lessen the patient's distress. Alongside each drip should be hung a container of 500 ml of 8·4 per cent sodium bicarbonate solution.

Abnormal heart rhythms may be avoided if the patient is resting and free of pain. The narcotic drugs already given may be supplemented by a sedative such as diazepam (Valium) up to 10 mg three times a day depending on the patient's tolerance. This does not produce a fall in blood pressure and cardiac output as happens with some barbiturates.

It is usual to give oxygen to all patients in the early stages. Six to eight litres per minute are usually given, either by double nasal catheter (Figure 23) or by face mask (see Figure 79). The oxygen is given because it has been found that, after myocardial infarction, the blood is more alkaline (pH over 7·4) than normal and there is a lower arterial pressure of oxygen. This may precipitate abnormal rhythms which do not respond to treatment until oxygen has been given. If oxygen by catheter or mask has no effect, it may be necessary to use a respirator.

The use of anticoagulants is still controversial. There is no evidence that long-term anticoagulants are of value. Some doctors use these short-term to prevent the formation of thrombus in the ventricles and in the peripheral veins, which may endanger life if an embolus from them blocks an artery in the brain, lungs or leg, etc. If a patient is likely to be confined to bed for a week or more, heparin has an immediate anticoagulant effect and may be given in continuous intravenous infusion or in six-hourly intramuscular injections. The dose is usually about 40 000 units in each 24 hours. Warfarin may be started at the same time, the heparin being discontinued after 48 hours. The warfarin is discontinued when the patient is up and about. There is now some evidence that low doses of subcutaneous heparin (5000 units, two or three times daily) are just as effective, and much less dangerous.

In general treatment, bed rest, usually for five to seven days depending on the severity of the infarction is usual. The recumbent position may be necessary until the pain and shock have subsided, when the semi-reclining or sitting position is suitable. The patient does not sit out

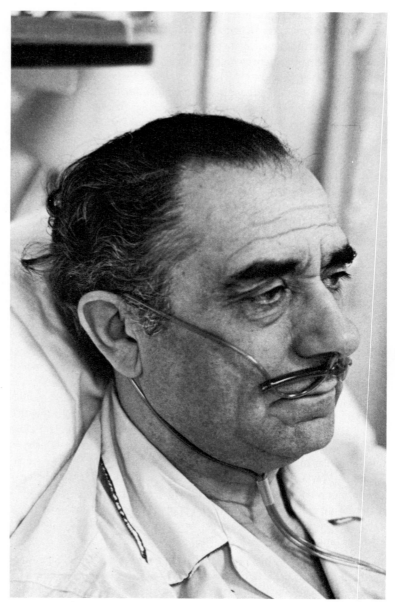

Figure 23 Double nasal catheter

in a chair until back in the general ward; after five to seven days of this, walking is permitted, increasing the amount each day. Patients should be able to negotiate a flight of stairs before they are discharged from the hospital after sixteen to twenty-one days.

The diet should be light, consisting of fluids only for the first few hours, and then a diet of about 1600 calories a day. Smoking is forbidden for the first few days and the patient should be encouraged to stop smoking.

It does not matter if the patient has no bowel motion for a day or two. However, a bedside commode is often more convenient and less strain than a bed-pan and, if necessary, a Dulcolax suppository or an enema may be given. Visitors are encouraged after the pain and shock has subsided, but only for a few minutes at a time.

The Coronary Care Unit

It is an increasing practice to treat patients with myocardial infarction in a special *Coronary Care Unit*. This has been found to considerably reduce the number of deaths involved. Indeed, specialized units for a variety of conditions are likely to become more numerous in the future.

Ideally, the Coronary Care Unit should be specially designed, although older wards may sometimes be converted quite successfully. From four to ten large single cubicles are needed, arranged so that the patients can all be seen from a central station yet cannot see each other (Figure 24). Access from the back of each cubicle should be possible so that, in cases of cardiac arrest, a patient can easily be removed while still in bed without alarming the other patients. A special treatment room and other rooms will be necessary for admission, relatives, doctors, nurses, secretary, records, equipment and linen. The patients' rooms should all have piped oxygen and suction and eight adequately earthed electrical outlets. All wiring in the neighbourhood of the unit must be shielded, and emergency electrical supplies must be available.

The beds should have no springs but a solid base with a plastic foam mattress to facilitate cardiac compression and the use of X-ray equipment. The bed head should be easily removable.

Equipment
Equipment (Figure 25) should be kept off the floor as much as possible. There should be continuous display of the electrocardiogram on an oscilloscope screen, and the heart rate shown on a meter both at the bed head and at the central station. The right atrial pressure can also be

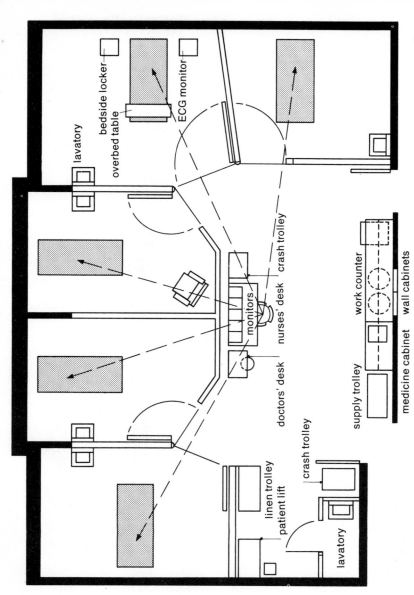

Figure 24 Plan of a Coronary Care Unit

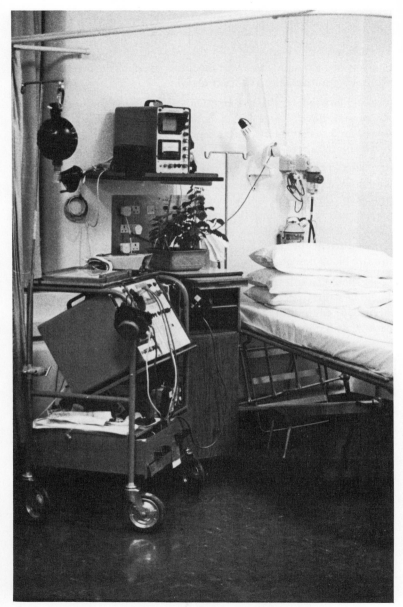

Figure 25 Special equipment in a Coronary Care Unit

continuously displayed using a simple manometer connected to a catheter whose tip is in the superior vena cava or the right atrium.

An alarm is usually connected with the pulse-rate meter and will trigger at a too low or a too rapid rate. This should be visible at the bed head and both visible and audible at the central station.

It should be possible to record an electrocardiogram at the bedside. This may be done directly from the oscilloscope. Various automatic systems may be used so that the electrocardiogram is recorded whenever anything triggers off the alarm. Alternatively, a memory tape can be included so that one can review the electrocardiogram of the previous few seconds.

More sophisticated measurements may be displayed, such as the pulmonary arterial pressure, systemic arterial pressure, respiration or temperature. But these may not help the management of the patient. Soon it may be possible to routinely record these things without having to puncture arteries or veins. For example, ultrasonic waves can be used to measure blood flow and blood pressure.

There should be at least two d.c. defibrillators in a unit, one of which should be battery operated and easily portable. Battery-operated pacemaking equipment is also needed, together with a portable X-ray machine with image intensification and a television screen. These are to facilitate the insertion of intracardiac electrodes. Other items of equipment needed are airways, endotracheal tubes, laryngoscopes, manual breathing bags with masks and apparatus for intermittent positive pressure respiration.

Coronary Care Units should be self-contained but preferably near to Intensive Therapy Units and to the wards into which the patients will eventually be discharged. These units demand skilled nursing attention, but give great satisfaction from the added responsibility and the direct involvement in the saving of life.

The admission of patients
All patients with chest pain thought to be due to myocardial infarction should be admitted to the unit. Most deaths occur in the first few hours so all patients should stay at least 72 hours, and preferably one week, although longer will be needed if complications occur.

The success of coronary care is largely dependent on the nursing staff. As well as general nursing, and the important relationship with the patient, the qualified nurse has a number of specialized duties. In many cases, she will be taught to initiate some treatment, giving drugs into the intravenous line:

heroin or morphine for pain
perphenazine for nausea
atropine for hypotension associated with bradycardia
lignocaine for ectopic beats, or other abnormal rhythms.

She must also know the drugs used in cases of cardiac arrest and prepare them by drawing them up into carefully labelled syringes ready for instantaneous use. She will also need to observe the oscilloscope, record electrocardiograms, record right-sided venous pressure either from a neck vein or from a manometer, record blood pressures, record the urinary output, watch the patient's general condition and listen for the tell-tale crepitations in the lungs which indicate left-sided heart failure. She may be taught to use the d.c. defibrillator. She should also know how to carry out external cardiac massage, mouth-to-mouth resuscitation, and know how to use the Ambubag. In addition, she should be taught how to pass an endotracheal tube and how to use mechanical ventilators.

After care
When a patient leaves the special unit for a general ward he is usually well on the way to recovery. However, careful observation is still necessary, since an appreciable number of late and often quite unexpected complications can occur. For example, late ventricular fibrillation is not uncommon. But if all goes well, the patient should be sitting out of bed after a few days and beginning to walk in about ten days. Most patients can leave the hospital in three weeks, but several weeks of programmed convalescence are then needed. However, this must not be overdone for, if the patient is not back at work after three months, there is a 50 per cent chance that he will never work again and, if six months elapse, he will certainly not go back at all. Normal activity helps most patients. Some need treatment for angina and a very few for persistent heart failure. Many patients lead a normal, active life for years before there is any recurrence.

Cardiac arrest

If the patient has collapsed and lost consciousness and the carotid pulse cannot be felt readily, then the circulation is inadequate and cardiac arrest has occurred (Figure 26). Respiration soon ceases, and the pupils dilate. No time should be wasted, and treatment must be initiated immediately. Although it is true that it takes three or four minutes before the lack of blood causes irreversible brain damage, the survival of the patient is closely related to the speed with which the cardiac arrest is dealt with. In dealing with any cardiac arrest, there are five important points to be remembered.

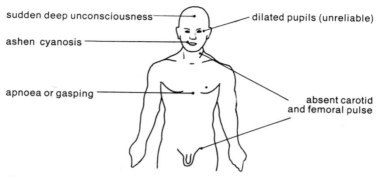

sudden deep unconsciousness

dilated pupils (unreliable)

ashen cyanosis

apnoea or gasping

absent carotid and femoral pulse

Figure 26 Signs of cardiac arrest

1 Never hesitate if in doubt, but act immediately. Do not wait to listen with a stethoscope, seek expert advice or send for an electrocardiogram.

2 The pupils must not be relied upon as a sign of cardiac arrest.

3 The patient must not be moved from his bed to the floor.

4 Cardiac massage must not be interrupted for longer than is absolutely necessary during attempts to restore heart action.

5 Electrical activity of the heart must not be confused with its mechanical activity. A pulse must be felt, not just an ECG complex seen.

If the patient is in a Coronary Care Unit and the oscilloscope shows ventricular fibrillation, electrical defibrillation must be performed immediately by the nurse or doctor who has observed the 'arrest'. If the patient is not attached to an oscilloscope, action must be taken until it is discovered whether asystole or ventricular fibrillation is the cause. This action can be summarized as follows:

1 A blow over the heart with a clenched fist may start the heart again, or rapid regular blows or even taps may keep it going. Elevating the patient's legs may help to increase the venous return and even start the heart again.

2 The alarm must be sounded and help summoned – the 'crash call'.

compressions/minute

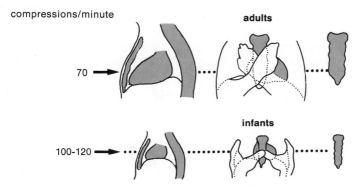

Figure 27 External cardiac massage in adults and infants.
Mid-sternal compression is important in infants to avoid liver rupture

3 External cardiac massage (Figure 27) must be started. This is hard
work, and relays may be needed. The hands are placed one on top of the
other, with the heel of the underneath hand over the lower sternum
(Figure 28). The sternum is then depressed rhythmically and forcefully

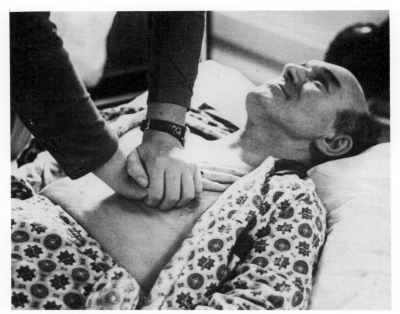

Figure 28 External cardiac compression

about 70 times per minute. In infants, much less force is needed, the thumbs at mid-sternal level (to avoid rupture of the liver) being sufficient (Figure 27). A more rapid rate of over 100 times per minute is necessary. If it is effective, the carotid and femoral pulses will be felt, and the pupils will become smaller.

4 Ventilation must be started at the same time. The neck is extended and the jaw pulled forward to stop the tongue falling back and obstructing the airway (Figure 29). If no equipment is available, mouth-to-mouth ventilation may be started. The operator pinches the patient's nose, puts his mouth over the patient's mouth and forces in air to inflate the patient's lungs. A handkerchief may be used between the mouths, although more satisfactory is a *Brook's airway* which has a mouthpiece for patient and operator. Usually one chest inflation is alternated with five cardiac compressions but this may not be possible if there is only one operator. An airway tube and an Ambu bag, with oxygen if available, is even better and easier to use. If the situation is prolonged, an endotracheal tube should be inserted and ventilation continued with oxygen through an Ambu bag. If the problem is not rapidly resolved, an artificial respirator may be needed, and sometimes a tracheostomy. If the patient is in a Coronary Care Unit, an endotracheal tube can be inserted as soon as possible and this is the best way of ensuring a proper airway.

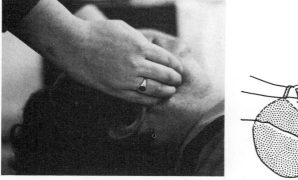 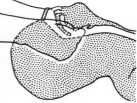

Figure 29 Maintenance of the airway.
Removal of the pillow and extension of the head clears the airway, and elevation of the jaw further improves it

5 Severe acidosis occurs quickly, so 200 mEq of sodium bicarbonate (200 ml of an 8·4% solution) should be given intravenously at once. More can be given later if necessary.

6 By this time the oscilloscope will have been attached to the patient and the rhythm identified. If it is ventricular fibrillation, electrical defibrillation with a d.c. shock is used at once. A large electric shock through the heart causes it to stop, but myocardium has an inherent rhythmic character so that it rapidly begins to beat again. The brief respite gives it the chance to recommence in its normal sinus rhythm, which fortunately it usually does. A d.c. shock will also terminate most rapid rhythms, so patients who lose consciousness with a rapid heart rate should be given treatment with d.c. shock immediately.

The defibrillator machine (Figure 30) delivers an electric shock. Usually about 300–400 Joules (watt-seconds) are needed to terminate ventricular fibrillation. Supraventricular tachycardia requires a much smaller charge

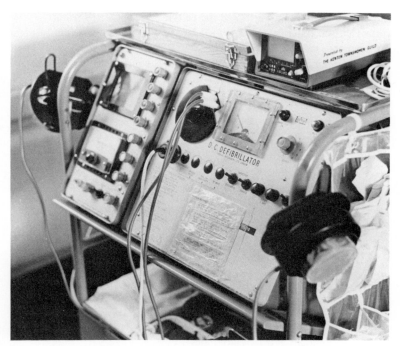

Figure 30 A resuscitation trolley with a d.c. defibrillator

and, in this case, there is less urgency and the shock should be synchronized with the R wave. The machine is switched on and allowed to build up the charge in its capacitance system. Electrode jelly should be applied liberally to the 'paddles' of the machine, the right upper chest and the left axilla of the patient. Care should be taken that the jelly is not smeared right across the patient's chest, and there should be none on the hands of the operator. Everyone but the operator should stand well back from the patient and the operator should not be touching the bed. With the paddles firmly in place (Figure 31), the switch is depressed and the patient convulses as the charge passes through his chest. Then the paddles are removed and the oscilloscope checked. If sinus rhythm has not returned, a further shock is given immediately. Lignocaine reduces cardiac irritability, and may be given to help. Repeated failure suggests that so much muscle has died that recovery is not possible.

If the oscilloscope indicates asystole rather than ventricular fibrillation, and the electrocardiogram records a straight line, the outlook is not good. A thump on the chest may start the heart but, if not, ventricular fibrillation must be induced, and then a d.c. shock given to restore sinus rhythm. Calcium chloride (5–10 ml of a 1 per cent solution intravenously) may achieve this end; if it is ineffective it may be repeated after a few minutes. Adrenaline (5–10 ml of a 1 in 10 000 solution) or

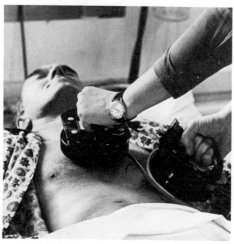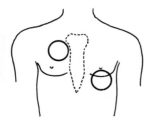

Figure 31 Positions of paddle electrodes

isoprenaline (0·1–0·2 mg) may be given intravenously or injected directly into the heart. If this does not work, pacing with the usual electrode or a 'stab' electrode straight into the heart may be tried.

Cardiogenic shock

Patients with cardiogenic shock have a cold sweating skin, low pulse volume, mental agitation, confusion or even coma, oliguria or anuria, continued ischaemic pain and an increased tendency to dangerous dysrhythmias and asystole. The risk of death is very high. Some deaths are inevitable because of the large amount of heart muscle that has died.

If treatment is to be successful, it must start as soon as the diagnosis is made. These patients have intense constriction of their peripheral blood vessels, the body's way of attempting to keep the blood pressure up. However, drugs which simply raise the blood pressure are of no use. If the patient looks and feels well and warm, and is excreting a reasonable amount of urine, it does not matter how low the blood pressure is. If the low blood pressure is associated with bradycardia, with or without shock, this may be corrected with an injection of atropine to counteract the excessive vagal activity, or by raising the legs to increase the venous return to the heart.

The constriction of the peripheral blood vessels may be counteracted by giving *phenoxybenzamine* in the intravenous drip in a single dose of 1 mg/kg over a two-hour period, the effect lasting for several days. Steroids such as *methyl prednisolone* (30 mg/kg) have a similar action. These drugs open up the peripheral circulation, and also allow blood to leave the pulmonary circulation and pass into the systemic circulation, thus easing any pulmonary oedema. But to maintain the blood pressure, more fluid is required, so 200 ml increments of 5 per cent dextrose solution are given. This treatment is repeated unless the right atrial pressure exceeds 12 cm, when further increments are withheld, and dixogin and diuretics given. A catheter is always kept in place in the bladder to show any increase in the passage of urine as perfusion of blood through the kidneys increases. This is important, for the first evidence of possible success is usually that the patient begins to pass urine.

In addition, isoprenaline, which has a direct stimulant action on the heart, may be given slowly with dextrose (4 mg isoprenaline in 500 ml dextrose), often with lignocaine as well, to prevent the abnormal rhythms that isoprenaline may cause. Ventilation with a respirator may also be helpful in the shock state. These techniques have been claimed to increase survival rates to 80 per cent instead of the more usual 20 per cent.

Other ways of assisting the circulation in shock are being tried. Blood has been pumped from a catheter in the left ventricle to the femoral artery. Also, helium-filled balloons have been passed through the femoral artery into the aorta, and blood forced along the circulation by alternately inflating and deflating them.

Surgical treatment is also being carefully studied. The infarcted area has been successfully removed (*infarctectomy*) allowing the remaining muscle to function properly, without having to support dead muscle as well. Multiple venous grafts to bypass the blocked vessels have been performed even in the shocked state, with good results.

If there is a complication such as a rupture of the interventricular septum, or of a papillary muscle with severe mitral regurgitation, or cardiac tamponade the surgeon may be able to help. However, many of these patients are so seriously ill that they die.

Summary of nursing points

The coronary circulation is one of the most important systems of blood transportation in the body. The reason for its importance is that it supplies the heart muscle with oxygen and nutrients, and removes its waste products. Without this, the circulation as a whole would cease. Therefore, any obstruction of the vessels that constitute this system, or of their tributaries, can produce serious (if not fatal) results for the patient.

The nurse must understand the coronary circulation, its design and functions. She should appreciate the main pathological conditions which are associated with the coronary vessels, and their clinical manifestations, together with the investigations and treatment of the patient.

The nursing care of the patient with myocardial infarction is important in his recovery. It must include the basic care and comfort of the patient, such as nursing position, his toilet and the carrying out of prescribed treatment conscientiously. The nurse must also record any variations in pulse, blood pressure, respiration, fluid balance and pain. Her role must also include the mental and emotional support of the patient.

The nurse must understand the predisposing causes of disease of the coronary vessels, and be knowledgeable in counselling the patient, as necessary, on his care and management. She should be able to explain about the taking of certain drugs, and about dietetic and social measures, which are important in enabling him to lead a reasonable life. She should appreciate the principles of specialized nursing care as practised in a Coronary Care Unit, must understand the use and maintenance of special apparatus, and be thoroughly conversant with the principles and method of application of emergency resuscitation, should the patient go into cardiac arrest.

Chapter 4

Abnormal rhythms and conduction

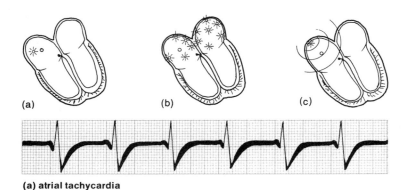

(a) atrial tachycardia

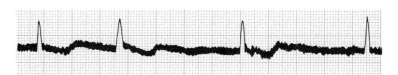

(b) atrial fibrillation

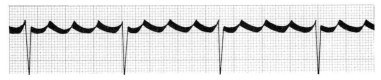

(c) atrial flutter

Figure 32 Electrocardiograms of supraventricular tachycardias; the origin of the electrical impulses are indicated on the accompanying heart diagrams

After myocardial infarction, minor abnormalities in heart rhythm are often followed by major abnormalities, such as ventricular fibrillation or asystole resulting in death. The skilled nurse should be able to detect these abnormalities on the oscilloscope as soon as possible, and initiate treatment. If at all possible, an electrocardiogram should be taken as a record.

Supraventricular tachycardias

These are unduly rapid heart beats, the impulse arising from anywhere between the sino-atrial and atrioventricular nodes. *Sinus tachycardia* is a regular rhythm of over 100 beats per minute and usually needs no treatment. *Atrial tachycardia* (Figure 32a) is somewhat similar, but the pacemaker is somewhere in the atria themselves and not in the sinus. On the electrocardiogram the P waves are unusual in shape and direction. The ventricles may respond to each atrial impulse, or block may occur, the ventricles responding to every second impulse. This often occurs in digoxin overdosage. In *nodal tachycardia*, the impulse arises from the atrioventricular node. The P waves are abnormal in direction and are close to the QRS complex, either before or after it or lost within it. In *atrial fibrillation* (Figure 32b), the atria 'shimmer' in an irregular manner, and are ineffectual as a pump. The atrioventricular node is bombarded with impulses, and responds in an irregular way. This very important and common dysrhythmia is mostly easily recognized by the complete irregularity of pulse, both in time and volume. On the electrocardiogram, the P wave is replaced by coarse or fine 'f' waves, and the QRS complexes occur irregularly and rapidly. *Atrial flutter* (Figure 32c) is a less common condition than fibrillation. In this, there is a regular atrial beat of about 300 per minute. The ventricles cannot respond as fast as this so they respond to each second, third or fourth impulse, but beating quite regularly. On the electrocardiogram, the P wave is replaced with saw-toothed waves.

Atrial tachycardia, nodal tachycardia and atrial flutter may respond temporarily or permanently to simple massage of the carotid sinus (Figure 33). This lies at the level of the upper border of the thyroid cartilage. Both carotid sinuses may be massaged in turn, but never together, as this may be dangerous.

Digoxin should be used to treat all the supraventricular tachycardias unless it is itself a possible cause of the abnormal rhythm. For among its toxic effects are abnormalities of heart rhythm, particularly atrial tachycardia with block. All degrees of heart block may also occur. The use of digoxin may be fatal if it is already producing toxic abnormal rhythms. Digoxin may be given by mouth or, if the patient is in heart failure and speed is essential, 0·5 mg may be given slowly intravenously. If this is not successful then the addition of propranolol by mouth may be helpful.

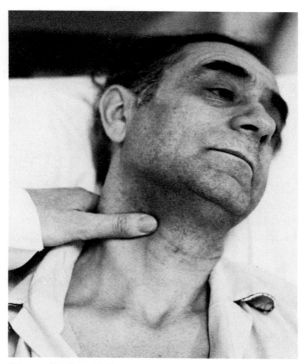

Figure 33 Carotid sinus massage

If the abnormal rhythm is not readily controlled or abolished, d.c. shock should be given under light anaesthetic. Usually only small energy levels are needed to re-establish sinus rhythm. The shock is triggered by the apparatus to coincide with the R wave of the electrocardiogram. This is to avoid the T wave and the danger of ventricular fibrillation (see below). But if ventricular fibrillation occurs, it can easily be corrected by a second shock.

Ventricular ectopic beats

These are also known as premature beats or premature ventricular contractions. This group of dysrhythmias may be seen in people with normal hearts. After myocardial infarction, they occur in about 80 per cent of patients, as a focus in a ventricle prematurely initiates a heart beat. The electrocardiogram shows an unusual, widened QRS complex, with a T wave in the opposite direction occurring early and followed by a compensatory pause (Figure 34a). If this pattern on the electrocardiogram occurs in runs of three or more (by definition *ventricular tachycardia*), or more often than one in ten beats or is very near the preceding T wave, the patient needs treatment. If the ectopic beat actually coincides with the T wave of the previous complex, a very dangerous situation is present and the ventricular ectopic beats may initiate *ventricular tachycardia* or *ventricular fibrillation*. The ectopic beats usually stop if 50–100 mg of lignocaine is given intravenously and repeated after 20 minutes. This can be followed with a lignocaine drip at a rate of 1–2 mg per minute to control possible recurrences. The rate can be controlled by the Coronary

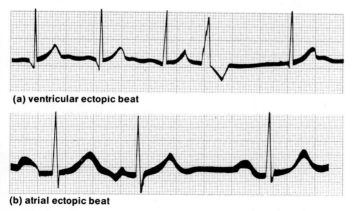

(a) ventricular ectopic beat

(b) atrial ectopic beat

Figure 34 Electrocardiograms of ectopic beats

Care nurse to the minimum that will prevent the abnormal rhythm. If this fails, procainamide may be tried, but it can cause a fall in blood pressure. It may be given intravenously at a rate of up to 100 mg per minute to a total of 1 g or by mouth in a dose of 500 mg each six hours. Other anti-arhythmic drugs such as phenytoin, propranolol, practolol, oxyprenolol or bretyllium may be used.

Atrial ectopic beats (Figure 34b) may also occur, but are less dangerous, although they may initiate atrial dysrhythmias. They have a normal QRS complex, but it occurs early and is followed by a compensatory pause. *Nodal ectopic beats* also occur with a normal QRS complex and P waves close to the QRS complex or lost in it.

Ventricular tachycardia

This is a dangerous rhythm which may lead to heart failure, greater shock and precipitate ventricular fibrillation. An irritable focus in the ventricle leads to ventricular contraction at a rate of over 140 per minute. It is usually a regular rhythm with a small pulse volume and a low blood pressure. The atria continue to beat at their normal rate. The electrocardiogram (Figure 35a) shows rapid broad QRS complexes like those of bundle branch block (see p. 71). There is a 60 per cent mortality, so ventricular tachycardia is always treated urgently. It often responds to lignocaine used as described above or to procainamide, phenytoin, propranolol, oxyprenolol or bretyllium. However, if not rapidly controlled, it should be abolished with a d.c. shock.

Ventricular fibrillation

There is chaotic ventricular activity with irregular impulses at a rate of over 300 per minute (Figure 35b). The ventricles have no pumping

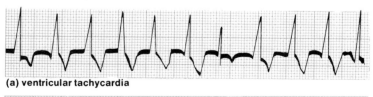
(a) ventricular tachycardia

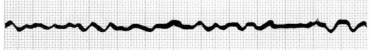
(b) ventricular fibrillation

Figure 35 Electrocardiograms of ventricular tachycardia and fibrillation

effect, and cardiac output is nil. The patient loses consciousness and rapidly dies if not treated. Fortunately, it can nearly always be corrected by d.c. shock (see p. 61).

Accelerated idioventricular rhythm

This describes a situation when the atria and ventricles beat independently, but the ventricular rate is quite rapid. The electrocardiogram looks like that of complete heart block (see p. 75) except that the ventricular rate is rapid. The QRS complexes are wide and bizarre and this rhythm can easily be mistaken for ventricular tachycardia. This is important, for it does not have the same bad prognosis and is usually transient.

Bundle branch block

If there is *left bundle branch block* (Figure 36a, Figure 37a), the electrical impulse cannot pass along the left bundle, and activation of the septum begins from the right instead of the left. The leads facing the left ventricle thus do not show the normal small Q wave, but a small R wave is shown. The right bundle is normal, so the right ventricle is activated next. This produces a small R wave in lead V1 and an S wave in lead V6. Finally, by a circuitous path, the left ventricle is activated, and this produces another R wave in lead V6 and an S wave in lead V1. Left bundle branch block is always an important disorder, and may be caused by non-specific fibrosis in older people, ischaemic heart disease and hypertension.

It is possible to identify electrocardiogram patterns due to block of either the left anterior or the left posterior branches and these are just as important as complete left bundle branch block.

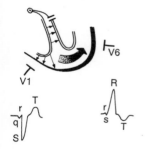

(a) left bundle branch block

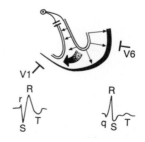

(b) right bundle branch block

Figure 36 Genesis of left and right bundle branch blocks

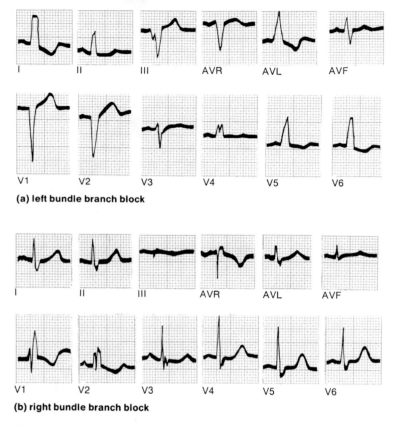

(a) left bundle branch block

(b) right bundle branch block

Figure 37 Electrocardiograms of left and right bundle branch blocks

In *right bundle branch block* (Figure 36b, Figure 37b), the septum is activated normally, so lead V6 shows a small Q wave and lead V1 a small R wave, as normal. Then the left ventricle is depolarized, resulting in the normal pattern of a tall R wave in lead V6 and a deep S wave in lead V1. Then the right ventricle contracts late and, because it is not opposed by the left ventricle, there is a big R wave in lead V1 and a deep S wave in lead V6. Right bundle branch block may be caused by non-specific fibrosis in older people and is occasionally seen in apparently healthy people. It occurs in acute pulmonary embolism (usually temporary), ischaemic heart disease, right ventricular hypertrophy from any cause, or in atrial septal defect, although then more often in a partial form.

Heart block

All heart muscle has a marked rhythmic property. The sino-atrial node initiates impulses at the rate of about 70 per minute, the atrioventricular node at about 60 and the bundle of His at about 50. The ventricular muscle itself has a rhythmic character, but its rate may be as low as 30. The part with the highest rate will initiate the heart beat and this is usually the sino-atrial node.

In *sino-atrial block*, the normal impulse completely fails to arise from the sino-atrial node, so that a complete heart beat is missed out ('dropped beat'). The electrocardiogram (Figure 38a) will show one PQRST complex completely missing, the next occurring in the expected place. Sino-atrial block may occur in the normal heart, in rheumatic carditis, after a myocardial infarction or from digoxin poisoning.

Sinus arrest occurs when the sinus node fails completely. No P waves are seen on the electrocardiogram and, after a variable interval, another 'pacemaker' will take over, usually the atrioventricular node, but sometimes a lower site. If this occurs after a myocardial infarction, it may be corrected with intramuscular atropine.

If there is a defect in conduction from the atria to the ventricles, *atrioventricular block* is said to be present. There are three degrees. In *first degree A–V block*, all the impulses reach the ventricles, but there is a delay in transmission resulting in the PR interval on the electrocardiogram being prolonged beyond its normal 0·20 seconds (Figure 38b). This is found quite commonly in rheumatic carditis, digitalis poisoning and myocardial infarction. It may progress to a higher degree of block or vanish spontaneously.

In *second degree A–V block*, some complete heart beats are lost ('dropped beats'). There are two types:

1 With a fixed A–V relationship (Figure 38c). Regularly or irregularly, the P wave will not be followed by a QRS complex. At the pulse, a beat will be missed altogether. Often there is a regular relationship so that every second or third beat is missed and it is referred to as a 'two to one' or a 'three to one' block.

2 With the *Wenckebach phenomenon*. In this variety, conduction through the conducting system becomes increasingly prolonged until a complete beat is dropped. This pause allows the conducting tissue time to recover, and then the cycle begins all over again. The electrocardiogram

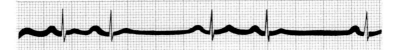

(a) sino-atrial block

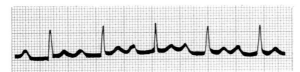

(b) first-degree heart block

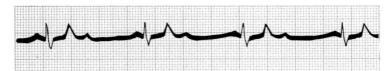

(c) second-degree heart block – two to one

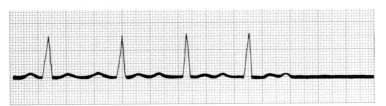

(d) second-degree heart block of Wenckebach type

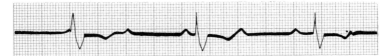

(e) complete heart block

Figure 38 Electrocardiograms of heart blocks

(Figure 38d) shows a P R interval getting longer with each successive beat until finally one P wave is not followed at all by a QR S complex, and then the cycle begins again. Often it is regular so that each third or fourth beat is lost. If it is each third beat that is lost, it gives rise to 'coupling' in which the heart beats occur in pairs followed by a pause. This is easily felt at the wrist.

Second degree heart block may occur in rheumatic or diphtheritic carditis, in digitalis overdosage and in ischaemic heart disease. If, after a myocardial infarction, the slow rate of second degree heart block is embarrassing the heart, treatment may be needed. Atropine may stop it, isoprenaline may increase the heart rate, or the heart may need to be paced artificially.

Third degree A–V block (Figure 38e) is known as complete heart block.

Complete heart block

In complete heart block, all the impulses from the atria are blocked and none reach the ventricles. The ventricles are then activated by a 'pacemaker' at a level lower than the block, either from within the conducting tissue or in the ventricles themselves. The lower down it is, the slower will be the heart rate.

The patient will have a slow, regular pulse of about 30 to 40 beats per minute. In the neck, venous 'a' waves may be seen occurring at a normal rate because the atria are contracting normally, but every now and again a 'cannon' wave will be seen. This occurs when the right atrium contracts while the tricuspid valve is closed, so the blood cannot get into the right ventricle and shoots up the jugular veins. On *auscultation* (listening), it will be found that the first heart sound changes in loudness because of the varying times of atrial contraction in relationship to filling of the ventricles. The cusps of the mitral and tricuspid valves at the beginning of systole are in varying positions. The further they have to travel to close, the louder is the first heart sound.

The electrocardiogram (Figure 38e) shows P waves occurring at a normal rate and QR S complexes occurring at a much slower rate, there being no regular relationship between the two. If atrial fibrillation or sinus arrest is also present, as may well happen in older patients, P waves will not be seen at all and there will be no venous or cannon waves in the neck.

The patient may complain of nothing at all, or simply of tiredness or breathlessness because of the poor cardiac output. He may go into frank heart failure as a result. If he already has angina or intermittent *claudication* (cramp-like pain in the legs, see p. 185), this may become worse. However, the most important complaint is that of attacks known as *Stokes–Adams attacks.*

In these attacks, the patient may just suddenly feel dizzy, have a convulsion or even suddenly lose consciousness. After ten to thirty seconds, during which time he will be pulseless, pale and cyanosed, he will regain consciousness and his face will flush as the circulation starts up again. These attacks are caused by short bouts of asystole (no heart beats) or ventricular fibrillation. They may occur frequently or infrequently, but sooner or later one will be prolonged and the patient will die. In most instances, the attacks end spontaneously, but no one should assume this will automatically be the case. A blow over the sternum with the clenched fist will often start the heart again. If it does not do so, the situation should be treated as cardiac arrest, and the appropriate procedure started (see p. 57).

The most common cause of complete heart block in elderly people is non-specific fibrosis in the conducting tissue. Many of these patients have good coronary circulations, so treatment of the condition is very worthwhile. Complete heart block may occur in ischaemic heart disease, particularly after a myocardial infarction, but if the patient survives the infarction, the heart block usually disappears. However, a few persist and need long-term treatment. There is a congenital form, but usually it has quite a rapid ventricular rate of about 60 beats per minute. Complete heart block may occur in rheumatic or diphtheritic carditis and as a complication of cardiac surgery. It is sometimes seen in aortic stenosis when the calcium from the valve has extended into the conducting tissue, and may also result from digitalis poisoning.

Treatment
Patients with complete heart block and symptoms, especially those with Stokes–Adams attacks, should be treated as soon as possible.
Stokes–Adams attacks may be abolished by giving long-acting isoprenaline (Saventrine) 15–60 mg three times a day.

However, too much effort should not be made to increase the ventricular rate, for there is considerable risk of causing ventricular arhythmias and death. It is preferable to use an artificial pacemaker. If this is to be used for only a short while, as in myocardial infarction or in the emergency

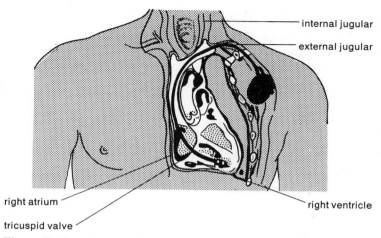

internal jugular

external jugular

right atrium

right ventricle

tricuspid valve

Figure 39 The placement of a pacemaker electrode in the right ventricle

treatment of frequent Stokes–Adams attacks, then an external battery-operated pacemaker will suffice. If long-term treatment is needed, an implanted pacemaker must be used.

The pacemaker consists of a wire electrode passed through the jugular vein (Figure 39) or a vein in the arm into the right atrium, through the tricuspid valve to the apex of the right ventricle, where it is firmly implanted. The other end is connected to a generator which supplies the pulses. This is usually quite small, contains its own batteries and is buried beneath the skin, usually in the axilla. Usually nowadays it works only when the patient's heart fails to generate an impulse, thus supplementing the heart to give a normal heart rate (*demand pacemaker*). The batteries last about two years, and then a small operation is carried out to replace the unit. However, the pacemaker needs regular checks which are carried out at special clinics. There are other more sophisticated varieties of pacemaker which carry out sequential pacing, stimulating the atrium first, followed by the ventricle, or which use the P wave of the electrocardiogram to trigger the pacemaker. Also, radioactive sources for the batteries are being developed which may have a life of about ten years. Another way to avoid the minor operation of replacing the unit is to fix the electrodes directly to the heart and initiate the impulses by an external battery-operated induction coil. Many doctors now believe that all patients with permanent heart block should have an artificial pacemaker inserted.

Atrioventricular dissociation

In complete heart block, the atria and the ventricles are dissociated. However, atrioventricular dissociation may occur without any organic block in the conducting tissue, for example with digoxin overdosage or after a myocardial infarction. It is important to recognize this as it does not have the same sinister significance that complete heart block has. Most of the time, the atria and the ventricles beat quite independently of each other, each having their own regular rhythm. However, every now and again an irregularity takes place when a normally conducted beat occurs. This happens because the ventricle is not refractory and accepts the impulse from the sino-atrial node and the atrium. This is called a 'capture beat' (Figure 40), the sino-atrial node having 'captured' the ventricle. It requires no special treatment unless it is due to digoxin, in which case the drug should be stopped.

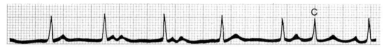

Figure 40 Electrocardiogram of atrioventricular dissociation; the beat labelled C is the capture beat

Summary of nursing points

The cardiac cycle, its initiation, conduction, control and variations must be understood by every nurse. This is particularly important for the nurse who is working in the Coronary Care Unit, where an abnormal rhythm, if not readily detected, its significance appreciated and subsequent treatment effected, can lead to the death of the patient. Once the normal rhythm of the heart and pulse is understood, the nurse will find that variations are more readily detectable, particularly on the oscilloscope.

The common abnormal rhythms which the nurse may see are sinus tachycardia, nodal tachycardia, atrial tachycardia and atrial fibrillation, and, less often, ventricular fibrillation. She should appreciate the condition of heart block and its grade. Finally, a major role of the nurse is to detect these abnormalities and to initiate prompt treatment.

Chapter 5 High blood pressure

The complications of high blood pressure (*hypertension*) cause, directly or indirectly, the death of about 20 per cent of the population of the United Kingdom. Hypertension is extremely common and, if it is effectively controlled, the length of life is increased. Yet high blood pressure is very difficult to define, as pressures vary from person to person, and even in the same person at different moments and at different ages. The critical aspect of high blood pressure is the level of the diastolic pressure. In any case, the level of systolic pressure is often raised as people get older because of the loss of the normal elasticity of the large blood vessels. In younger people, this elasticity absorbs and levels out the high pressure at which blood is ejected from the left ventricle.

For clinical purposes, we can take the normal level of the blood pressure in an adult as 130 mmHg (millimetres of mercury) systolic pressure and 80 mmHg diastolic; this is usually written as 130/80, and there is an upper limit of 150/90. At birth, the pressure is about 80/60 and over the years gradually rises to the adult level.

Physiological control of the blood pressure

The distribution of blood to the various organs of the body is controlled by variation in the size of the blood vessels before capillary level is reached. These vessels have muscular walls and may be relaxed under nervous control, allowing more blood to flow, or contracted, allowing less blood to flow. But the demands of organs vary, and the distribution of the blood must be controlled. For example, someone running on a hot day after a large meal will need extra blood supplied to the muscles, gut and skin. Yet if all these vessels enlarged, the blood pressure would drop, and the brain and the heart would not get enough blood, with the possibility of dangerous consequences.

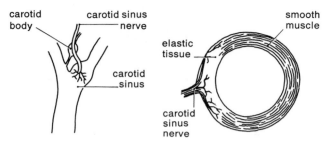

Figure 41 Carotid sinus stretch receptors

Where the common carotid artery divides into its internal and external branches, at the beginning of the internal branch, is a swelling called the *carotid sinus*. Here, and also in the aortic arch, are special nerve endings called *stretch receptors* (Figure 41). These respond to stretching of the arterial wall and thus continuously measure arterial blood pressure. The nerve fibres from the carotid sinus travel in the glossopharyngeal (ninth) cranial nerve and those from the aortic arch in the vagus (tenth) nerve to the centres in the medulla of the brain which regulate the cardiovascular system. These centres send out impulses to the heart and to the blood vessels all over the body via the vagus nerve and via the sympathetic nerve fibres. Stimulation of the vagus nerve will slow the heart, and stimulation of the sympathetic fibres will increase its rate.

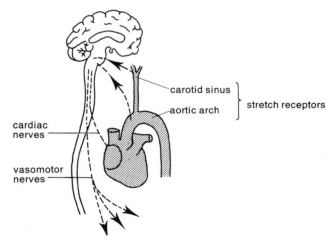

Figure 42 Control of arterial blood pressure

Stimulation of the sympathetic fibres will increase the force of atrial and ventricular contraction and a diminution will decrease it. Similarly, the degree of constriction or relaxation of the distant arterioles in various organs may be varied and so the flow may be varied. This variation of the size of the distant arteries will vary the peripheral resistance offered to the flow of blood and thus the arterial blood pressure (Figure 42). This peripheral control seems to be the most important mechanism in determining blood presssure, and is largely exercised in the skin and the gut, protecting vital organs such as the heart and the brain. This strict control mechanism keeps the arterial pressure within a reasonable range.

The measurement of blood pressure

Blood pressure is usually measured with a *sphygmomanometer* (Figure 43). This gives the pressure in millimetres of mercury, and is based either on

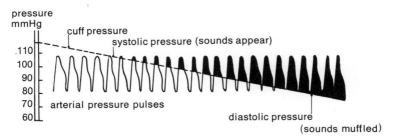

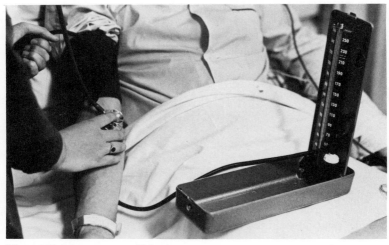

Figure 43 Measurement of blood pressure

the aneroid principle or on a column of mercury. The patient should be relaxed, and a cuff containing an inflatable rubber bag is wound firmly and evenly round his arm, the centre of the bag lying over the brachial artery, and the lower edge of the cuff just above the bend of the elbow. The cuff is then inflated with air by means of a rubber bulb, until the brachial pulse can no longer be felt. This is because the artery has been compressed and the systolic pressure is exceeded by the pressure in the cuff. The cuff is then slowly deflated until the brachial pulse reappears. The pressure at which this occurs equals the *systolic pressure*. The cuff is then inflated again and the process repeated, this time listening with a stethoscope to the sounds over the brachial artery. As the cuff is deflated, sounds are heart with each heart beat. The point at which these first appear is the systolic pressure. Deflation is continued and the sounds tend to get louder and louder, but then suddenly become muffled and finally disappear altogether. The pressure at the point where the sounds become muffled equals the *diastolic pressure*. In some patients there is a phase between systolic and diastolic pressure when sounds cannot be heard; this should be appreciated and the pulse used to indicate systolic pressure, in order to avoid inaccurate recordings. Blood pressure measurements are essential, not only in hypertension, but in many other conditions as well.

Hypertension

An abnormally high blood pressure leads to complications, which in turn lead to death. Treatment can lessen the incidence of these complications. The higher the diastolic pressure, the shorter the time the patient will live. It may even be that people who show unusually high blood pressures from emotional causes but have normal blood pressures at other times may expect shortened lives. There are four serious complications of hypertension. High blood pressure accelerates cerebral atherosclerosis and may result in *strokes* (cerebral thrombosis or haemorrhage). Heart failure may occur, at first on the left side, but eventually congestive heart failure will supervene. Hypertension, particularly the malignant form, may cause kidney failure and death from uraemia. Hypertension also accelerates coronary atheroma, so angina is common and death may occur from myocardial infarction.

Hypertension may be *malignant* or *benign*. If it is malignant, the diastolic pressure is usually 130 mmHg or more; there is papilloedema (see p. 85), retinal exudates and haemorrhages in the fundus of the eye, and characteristic histological changes occur in the kidney which may be seen in a biopsy or in a post-mortem specimen. The outlook is very poor and most sufferers die within a year if they are not treated. In all other cases, it is called benign hypertension in spite of the fact that many complications occur and it sometimes progresses to the malignant phase. Hypertension is more usefully divided into two groups, *primary or essential hypertension* and *secondary hypertension.*

Essential hypertension

This accounts for about 95 per cent of all cases of hypertension, yet no definite cause has been found. Inheritance, sex, race and environment may all play a part.

Secondary hypertension

There are very few cases of secondary hypertension, but there are many causes (Figure 44). Most patients with raised blood pressure should be carefully investigated in case they have secondary hypertension. There are a number of diseases which may cause this form of hypertension. The patient may have a renal disease. Patients with acute glomerular nephritis may have high blood pressure and this may lead to death, although most make a complete recovery. Chronic renal diseases such as the late stages of glomerular nephritis or pyelonephritis often lead to high blood pressure and its complications. Polycystic disease of the kidneys is a congenital disease in which both kidneys are enlarged from the cysts they contain. About 50 per cent of these patients have high blood pressure. *Stenosis* (narrowing) of the renal artery may be due to overgrowth of muscle in the wall of the artery, to atheroma, aneurysm formation or embolus, and can lead to hypertension. It may occasionally be cured by reconstruction of the diseased artery or removal of the kidney. In addition, a few patients with toxaemia of pregnancy may be left with persistent hypertension. This disease probably has a renal cause, but it is an unknown one. Oedema of the face and hands, high blood pressure and albuminuria occur, and may go on to fits and renal failure, when termination of the pregnancy may be necessary. However, in most patients the hypertension subsides.

The patient may have an endocrine disorder. Phaeochromocytoma is a tumour of the medulla of the adrenal gland, usually benign but occasionally malignant, which secretes noradrenaline and adrenaline and causes hypertension. The hypertension is often paroxysmal but may

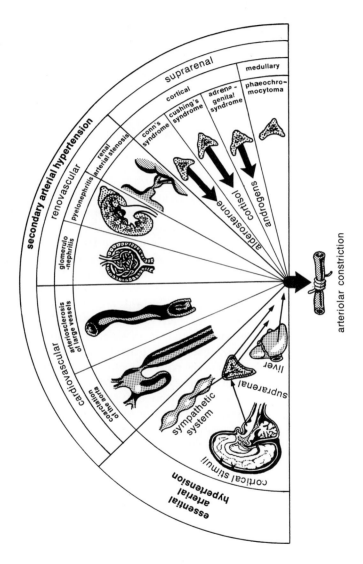

Figure 44 Causes of secondary hypertension

be permanent. The patients have attacks of headache, palpitations and sweating and are often thought to be neurotic. If the blood pressure is taken at these times, it is found to be raised. The hypertension can be corrected by giving them *phentolamine* intravenously, and this can be used as a test for the condition. The usual test is to estimate the amount of VMA (vanilmandelic acid) an end-product of adrenaline and noradrenaline metabolism, in the urine. Hypertension is one of the many features of Cushing's disease caused by overactivity of the adrenal cortex. A tumour in the adrenal cortex can cause the uncommon but correctable disease, *Conn's syndrome* (aldosteronism), in which hypertension is found. In this disease, excess aldosterone is secreted causing the patient to reabsorb sodium and to excrete abnormal amounts of potassium from the distal tubules in the kidney. The tumour should be removed if possible.

Other causes of hypertension are coarctation of the aorta (a congenital abnormality – see p. 139), collagen diseases such as polyarteritis nodosa and systemic lupus erythematosis, and diseases of the central nervous system such as bulbar poliomyelitis, encephalitis and an occasional intracranial tumour.

Symptoms
There are no symptoms which are due to the raised blood pressure itself, and the condition usually comes to light when it presents as one of its complications. It may be found during a routine examination, it may be first noticed in pregnancy, or the changes in the fundus of the eye may cause an optician to send the patient to his doctor. The blood pressure can be considerably raised for many years without the patient being aware of it.

On examination, the blood pressure will be found to be raised, the diastolic reading being over 90 mmHg. In the more severe cases, the apex beat will be forceful from left ventricular hypertrophy and an atrial sound may be heard; if the heart is failing, a third sound may be heard. Hypertension may be graded in severity by the changes seen with an ophthalmoscope in the fundus of the eye. The retinal arteries become narrowed and irregular and may constrict the veins where they cross them as they wind across the retina. In later stages haemorrhages of various kinds appear alongside the vessels. Exudates form and look like patches of cotton wool. Finally the head of the optic nerve may be seen to swell and become abnormally pink with blurred edges (*papilloedema*).

Hypertension may be divided into four grades of severity:

Grade 1 Irregular narrowing of the retinal arterioles.

Grade 2 Narrowing of arterioles and 'nipping' of the veins at the points where they cross.

Grade 3 Changes of 1 and 2 together with exudates and haemorrhages.

Grade 4 Papilloedema. The changes of 1 and 2 are always present and usually those of 3 as well. This indicates malignant hypertension.

Investigations
All patients with raised blood pressure should, ideally, be investigated for possible causes. Most patients will have *essential hypertension*, but the causes of some with secondary hypertension can be corrected. However, older patients, and those who have a strong family history of hypertension, may not justify such inconvenient and expensive investigation.

Clinical examination will decide the severity of the hypertension. The femoral pulses should always be felt for the characteristic poor volume and delayed impulse of coarctation of the aorta (see p. 139). Chest X-rays will show the size of the heart, which should not be much enlarged unless the heart is failing. An electrocardiogram may show some evidence of left ventricular hypertrophy in the more severe grades.

A midstream specimen of urine should be examined for albumin, which would suggest a renal cause, and for blood cells and organisms. It should be cultured and the finding of a bacterial infection would suggest pyelonephritis, although this often exists with no such evidence. The blood urea might be raised above 40 mg per cent if there is kidney involvement either as a cause or from damage done by the high blood pressure. The serum electrolytes should be estimated. In an aldosterone-secreting tumour, the potassium would be low and the chloride low with a raised or a normal sodium. A phaeochromocytoma secreting adrenaline or noradrenaline will excrete these in the urine in the form of VMA. If there is more than 6 mg VMA in a 24-hour specimen of urine, a phaeochromocytoma must be suspected.

The kidney structure and function may be examined by taking X-rays of the kidneys excreting an iodine-containing dye which is radio-opaque and is given into a vein. This is an *intravenous pyelogram*. Evidence of chronic pyelonephritis or of kidney disease on only one side may be found. If this and other tests suggest disease of a renal artery, a catheter can be passed from the femoral artery into the abdominal aorta to the level of the renal arteries, and dye injected. The X-ray pictures will show the anatomy of the blood supply to the kidneys and any evidence of obstruction in a renal artery. This is called *renal arteriography*.

Treatment
This is always necessary if there is malignant hypertension (grade 4 fundi) or if there is evidence of damage having already been done to the heart or kidneys. In young people, the finding of a raised blood pressure is enough to justify treatment but, in an old person with no symptoms and no evidence of damage, it is doubtful if this is the case, especially as the treatment may make them uncomfortable. Clearly, if a cause for the hypertension has been discovered, this must be treated.

Many drugs may be used in treatment. However, drug treatment requires careful consideration as not only do many of the more powerful drugs have unpleasant side effects, but treatment must be continued for the patient's lifetime. The doctor usually restricts himself to a few drugs and thoroughly learns their possibilities and combinations. However, new drugs are constantly being produced. There are a number of main groups of drugs:

1 Sedatives and tranquillizers may be very useful in the anxious patient and may even be all that is needed in the very mild cases.

2 The Rauwolfia group are derived from the root of the Indian plant *Rauwolfia serpentina* and deplete the body tissues of the hypertension-causing noradrenaline. Normally reserpine is used, given by mouth in doses of 0·25 mg once or twice a day.

3 Diuretics such as the thiazide group and frusemide (see p. 33) have a mild hypotensive action as well as their diuretic action. As well as lowering the blood volume, they may affect the muscular coat of the peripheral arteries and reduce arterial resistance, thereby lowering the blood pressure. They may be sufficient by themselves in mild hypertension, but are most often used to increase the effect of other hypotensive drugs. They tend to cause potassium depletion, so potassium supplements must be given.

4 Adrenergic blockers have been the most important development so far in the treatment of hypertension. There are four main types. The most useful at present is *methyldopa* (Aldomet) which prevents the manufacture in the body of noradrenaline and depletes the tissue stores of

adrenaline and noradrenaline although the exact mechanisms are uncertain. It is effective in severe hypertension, and may be given by mouth, 250 mg three or four times a day, increasing to as much as 750 mg four times a day if necessary. It may lead to sleepiness and cause a dry mouth, nasal congestion, retention of fluid and impotence. Haemolytic anaemia is not uncommon but is usually mild. *Guanethidine* (Ismelin) inhibits the adrenergic nerves of the sympathetic nervous system, blocks the release of noradrenaline, and reduces tissue stores. It takes some days to exert its full effect so it is started in a small dose by mouth (10 mg) and increased each five days until control is achieved – sometimes needing up to 500 mg a day. It need be given only once a day. It is more effective in the standing position, so blood pressure should be taken in that position. A disadvantage is that dizziness or even loss of consciousness may occur on getting up from a sitting or lying position (*postural hypotension*), and the patient should be warned of this. Other side-effects are diarrhoea, muscle pain or weakness and failure of ejaculation.

Bethanidine (Esbatal) resembles guanethidine but is not so long-acting and does not cause diarrhoea; however, it has the other disadvantages. It is started in a dose of 10 mg twice daily and increased each day. Often 100 mg daily will be needed. A drug very similar to bethanidine and used in the same dosages is *debrisoquine* (Declinax).

5 *Ganglion blockers* inhibit the transmission of all sympathetic and parasympathetic nervous impulses in the autonomic ganglia. These have so many disadvantages, that they are seldom used in treatment, except for the unusual hypertensive who fails to respond to other drugs and when intravenous therapy is needed to reduce blood pressure urgently.

6 *Propranolol* blocks certain receptors in the sympathetic nervous system and leads to a decrease in heart work and a reduction in peripheral resistance. It is used mostly for the treatment of angina and abnormal rhythms but is also used to treat hypertension, especially where they occur together. Very large doses of up to several grams a day may be needed. This drug is being increasingly used in treatment and has few of the undesirable side-effects.

7 *Clonidine hydrochloride* (Catupres) has a hypotensive effect equal to that of Aldomet, and does not lead to impotence or failure of ejaculation, although it may cause constipation. It seems to dilate the peripheral blood vessels and decrease peripheral resistance by a direct effect on the vasomotor centres in the brain. It may be started with 100 μg three times a day by mouth and increased on alternate days up to 4 or 5 mg daily.

Patients who need drug treatment will have to attend their doctor or clinic regularly. They should understand the reasons for the choice of drugs and why they must be continued in spite of unpleasant side-effects. They often like to know their blood pressure readings, and in some places are taught to take them themselves. There is much to recommend this practice.

If the hypertension is mild, treatment may start with reserpine (0·25 mg once or twice a day) or with a diuretic alone, perhaps cyclopenthiazide (0·5 g once or twice daily). It can be given in a tablet also containing potassium or with the potassium given separately, as there is a risk of potassium depletion.

If this does not work after a week or two or if the hypertension is more severe at the outset, a more powerful drug such as methyldopa may be started at a dose of 250 mg three times a day increasing at each visit to a maximum of 750 mg four times a day. However, before reaching this level, a diuretic added to the regime may increase the action of the methyldopa and also have a hypotensive action in its own right. A dose of 40 mg of frusemide a day can be used or 0·5–1·0 g of cyclopenthiazide. Potassium may also be needed.

If this fails, bethanidine, debrisoquine or guanethidine with or without diuretics are usually tried, and control is achieved by varying the combination. Three or even four drugs together may occasionally be necessary. Control means that the diastolic pressure is 100 mmHg or below.

In the early stages of severe hypertension, the level of blood urea must be watched. This is usually unaffected, but may fall or rise. It may rise and then flatten out to a new higher, but acceptable, level. However, occasionally it rises precipitously and treatment must be discontinued.

Urgent treatment
If hypertensive encephalopathy with fits or even coma in a hypertensive patient occurs, the blood pressure must be urgently reduced. This is also the case if hypertensive left ventricular failure fails to respond to aminophylline, morphine and oxygen. The patient is admitted to hospital immediately, and frequent blood pressure recordings are charted. Ganglion blockers such as pentolinium, 1 mg intravenously every five minutes, are usually given until the diastolic pressure is below 100 mmHg. Reserpine, (0·5–1·0 mg intravenously) may be equally effective. Once control is achieved, treatment is continued by mouth. More recently, diazoxide (300 mg intravenously) has been used and is most effective.

Summary of nursing points

The pressure exerted on the walls of the arteries by the blood coming from the left ventricle is known as *blood pressure*. The pressure produced during ventricular contraction is known as the *systolic pressure*; the pressure during ventricular relaxation is known as the *diastolic pressure*.

Various factors help to maintain normal blood pressure; these include the output of the heart during each contraction, the amount of blood in the circulation, the capillary resistance, the viscosity of the blood and the return of venous blood to the heart. Various diseases may cause hypertension, but most cases are of unknown cause. The nurse should understand the method of taking and recording blood pressure. She should also be aware of the clinical signs, investigations, complications and treatment of hypertension. The patient must be observed for signs of giddiness, difficulty in vision, headache, loss of appetite, changes in urinary output, bowel action and weight. The nurse must ensure that the treatment prescribed in respect of diet, rest and drugs is rigidly implemented. If the patient is prescribed complete bed rest, then everything must be done for him, including feeding, bathing and alteration of nursing position.

Chapter 6

Heart valve disease

A very useful guide to the conditions inside the heart may be obtained by listening to the heart sounds, a technique known as *auscultation* (Figure 45). This provides information particularly about the workings of the heart valves.

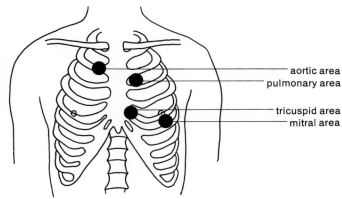

aortic area
pulmonary area

tricuspid area
mitral area

Figure 45 Sites of auscultation

The stethoscope

The stethoscope is used to listen to heart sounds and murmurs (Figure 46). It is a simple tube which conducts the sound waves from the patient's chest to the doctor or nurse's ear. There are usually two ends, one bell-shaped, which picks up low-pitched sounds, and one with a diaphragm stretched across its shallow, wide end which picks up the high-pitched sounds.

Heart sounds
First heart sound

This is caused by the closure of the mitral and tricuspid valves, as the pressures in the ventricles rise at the beginning of systole. It can be

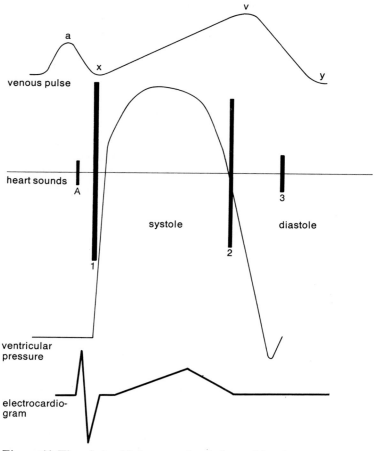

Figure 46 The relationship between electrical, arterial and venous pressure and sound events

timed by feeling the carotid artery pulse with one finger. The first heart sound coincides with this pulse. It may appear split into two components, because the left ventricle is more powerful than the right and raises its internal pressure more quickly, so that mitral valve closure occurs earlier.

Second heart sound

This is caused by the closure of the aortic and pulmonary valves as the pressure falls in the ventricles at the end of systole. This is normally split into two components, and the degree of splitting increases in inspiration and decreases with expiration. Not only does the aortic valve close before the pulmonary valve but, as the patient inspires, more blood is sucked into the right side of the heart; right-sided systole therefore takes longer, and the pulmonary valve closes even later.

Third heart sound

This occurs in early diastole and coincides with the period of diastole when the mitral and tricuspid valves have opened, and ventricular filling is rapid. It may be caused by muscular vibration. For no known reason, it occurs commonly in normal young people but in adults it is an important sign of heart failure or impending heart failure.

Fourth heart sound

This is also known as the atrial sound and is always abnormal. It occurs when the ventricle is diseased in some way and the atrium has to make a greater contribution to the filling of the ventricle. It occurs in late diastole, and may be right or left sided. It is probably a sound made by the ventricular muscle and caused by the reception into the ventricle of the blood driven out by the contracting atrium in late diastole. Although it does not occur in the normal heart, it does not have the serious significance that the third heart sound does in the adult.

Heart murmurs

The heart sounds mentioned are all transient, but heart murmurs continue for a longer time. If a heart murmur is very loud, it may be felt with the examining hand, and is known as a 'thrill'. Murmurs are due to undue turbulence of the blood as it passes through the heart. This may be caused by obstruction to the smooth flow of the blood or to its back flow (regurgitation) through a valve which normally would have been closed, but has become incompetent. Murmurs may be described by their occurrence in systole between the first and second heart sounds, or in diastole, between the second heart sound and the next first heart sound. They may be continuous and heard in both systole and diastole. They may vary in length, pitch or character, and these will help in deciding their cause.

It is necessary to listen all over the chest and to study many features of the sounds and murmurs before one can be sure from which valve they come. It is particularly useful to obtain an exact timing of sounds and

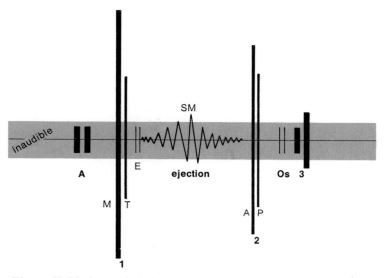

Figure 47 Ideal normal phonocardiogram.
A (atrial sound) represents the ventricular filling vibrations resulting from right and left atrial contraction. The first sound (1) comprises mitral (M) and tricuspid (T) components. The ejection vibrations (E) are followed by a physiological ejection systolic murmur (SM). The second sound (2) comprises aortic (A) and pulmonary (P) components. Os represents the opening of the tricuspid and mitral valves and is followed by rapid filling of the right and left ventricles (3 – third sound)

murmurs. The *phonocardiogram* (Figure 47) records heart sounds and murmurs on a graph, and the electrocardiogram or carotid pulse can be used to time them correctly.

Rheumatic heart disease
An important cause of heart disease and damage to heart valves is rheumatic heart disease, and this often causes disability and death. Rheumatic fever is less common than it used to be, and is now much milder. However, it is still common for children, and even young adults in their thirties, to get smouldering rheumatic fever and rheumatic carditis that is often difficult to diagnose, but leads to chronic rheumatic heart disease.

Rheumatic fever

This is likely to occur in a child who has a family history of rheumatic fever and lives in a poor social environment. About two or three weeks after the onset of a sore throat, he may suffer general malaise, loss of appetite, some fever, and vague aches in the limbs. Then, the typical arthritis begins, the joints involved becoming painful, hot, red and swollen. The larger joints are usually affected, one after the other. The small joints of the hands and feet are not often affected. Generally the arthritis disappears in a few weeks, even if it is not treated.

Nodules may be felt under the skin closely associated with tendons and joint capsules, particularly over the elbows, ankles, knees, and the back of the head. A rash of large pink circles (*erythema marginatum*) may be seen on the trunk. Inflammation of the heart (carditis) occurs in at least half of the patients, although not all will be left with permanent changes. Any or all of the tissues of the heart may be involved.

If *pericarditis* (see p. 158) is present, it is usually associated with *myocarditis* (see p. 166) and *endocarditis*. There may be chest pain and a pericardial friction rub or a pericardial effusion. There may also be changes in the electrocardiogram. Myocarditis is not easy to diagnose, but is probably present more often than is thought. It would be suggestive if the heart rate was fast, the heart was enlarged or heart failure developed which could not be explained by valve abnormalities. The electrocardiogram might show prolongation of the P R interval.

If murmurs are heard coming from the damaged endocardium of the heart valves, endocarditis is probably present. There may be mitral regurgitation (a long systolic murmur), aortic regurgitation (a diastolic murmur) and transient or persistent mitral diastolic murmurs which, over the years, may take on the characteristics of chronic mitral or aortic valve disease.

The cause of the rheumatic fever seems to be a sensitivity to the effects of infection with a particular streptococcal organism, group A βhaemolytic, but the exact mechanism is not known. Infection with this organism is common but only a few people get rheumatic fever.

Laboratory tests are helpful in diagnosis, but this is usually made clinically. The white blood count is usually raised to about 15 000 per cubic mm and the blood sedimentation rate (E S R) is high. The course of the disease may be followed by carrying out a series of E S R measurements. In a few cases, the streptococcus may be grown on a culture medium. The most usual evidence of the infection is given by a test which shows a high level of *antistreptolysin O* (A S O T) in the blood, which subsequently falls.

Treatment

The patient should have bed rest until evidence of activity has subsided, and the temperature, pulse rate and ESR have become normal. The carditis has probably then healed. There is no evidence that prolonged bed rest lessens the incidence of permanent valve damage. The patient is then encouraged gradually to resume normal activity. Usually a salicylate such as aspirin (not sodium salicylate as the sodium may lead to water retention and precipitate heart failure) is effective in a dose of 50–80 mg per kg daily in divided doses. This relieves the joint symptoms and signs, and will bring down the fever, but neither this nor steroids, which may also be used, seem to have any effect on the subsequent incidence of valve damage.

If the carditis is prolonged or very severe, prednisone, 40 mg daily in divided doses, gradually reducing to 5–10 mg daily over several weeks, is substituted. Heart failure, should it occur, is treated with digoxin and diuretics. Penicillin, for example procaine penicillin (600 mg units twice daily for seven days), should be given to eradicate any residual streptococcal infection.

Many patients make a good and rapid recovery, even if they were initially severely ill. However, some may be ill for months, and recurrent attacks are common. Very occasionally, the carditis and toxicity are so severe that the young patient fails to respond to treatment and dies. Pericarditis always heals and myocarditis usually does. However, many patients have permanent endocardial damage of the heart valves. The healing tissue becomes fibrous, contracts, and gradually produces valve abnormalities. Occasionally, there is persistent myocardial inflammation which may later contribute to heart failure. In very severe myocarditis, the mitral valve ring may enlarge greatly, leading to severe mitral regurgitation. This is particularly common in the virulent rheumatic fever seen in many tropical countries.

Prevention

Any patient who has had an attack of rheumatic fever should be given either penicillin V (125 mg by mouth twice a day) or, preferably, sulphadimidine (0·5 g twice a day) to prevent recurrent infection with streptococci and the risk of another attack of rheumatic fever. This prophylactic treatment should be continued well into adult life, to prevent the development of rheumatic carditis later.

Rheumatic chorea

This is also known as *Sydenham's chorea* or *St Vitus' Dance*. It is a neurological form of acute rheumatism, often with no clear history of any preceding streptococcal infection. The first sign is an insidious onset of violent, jerky purposeless movements in an otherwise healthy child. If it is confined to one side it is known as *hemichorea*. It can only be treated with sedatives and eventually the patient recovers. However, it frequently leads to valve damage and heart disease.

The mitral valve

The mitral valve (Figure 48) separates the left atrium and the left ventricle. It is most complex, both anatomically and in its mechanism. It is also very strong, for example, during a normal lifetime it will

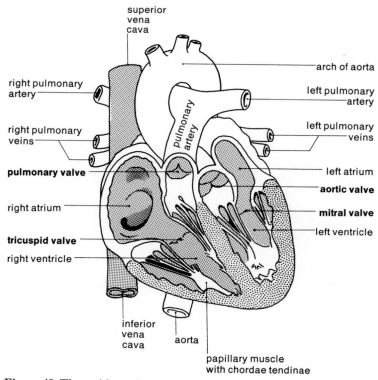

Figure 48 The positions of the heart valves

open and close some 2700 million times. It is enclosed in a fibrous ring
and has two cusps, the *anterior* (aortic) cusp and the *posterior* cusp. The
anterior cusp is much larger than the posterior. The edges of the cusps
are attached to strands of tendon known as the *chordae*, which are joined
to the two papillary muscles in the ventricles. The anterior cusp is
controlled by chordae from both muscles, but the posterior cusp by
chordae from only one of them. During systole, the chordae are tensed
by the papillary muscles, and this stops the cusps from ballooning into
the left atrium.

Mitral stenosis

Rheumatic heart disease has the effect of inflaming the cusps and, where
they meet while the valve is closed, they become adherent. Fibrosis occurs
and the remaining opening becomes much smaller. The normal valve
opens to 5 cm^2, but a severely diseased valve may open to no more than
1×0.5 cm. Moderate stenosis is well tolerated but severe obstruction
causes serious symptoms. The cusps of the valves tend to remain pliable
until later in life when they become rigid from fibrosis and calcification. In
a few cases, the chordae become fibrosed and shortened and the mitral
valve orifice becomes funnel-shaped.

The cardiac output is thus reduced because not enough blood can get
through the valve to the left ventricle and thus to the circulation. Changes
are also produced in the lungs. Because of the obstruction to flow, the
pressure in the left atrium and therefore in the pulmonary veins
increases. Acute pulmonary oedema may occur if the pressure rises
rapidly to more than 30 mmHg, thus exceeding the osmotic pressure in
the capillaries. More often, however, the pressure rises slowly over a period
of many years and fluid gradually exudes into the alveolar walls, with the
result that they thicken in compensation, and create a barrier which
protects the patient against pulmonary oedema. However, this also
stiffens the lungs, and makes the work of breathing more difficult, and
oxygenation of the blood less efficient.

The increased pressure in the pulmonary veins necessitates an increase
in pressure in pulmonary arteries and, therefore, in the right ventricle,
in order to maintain forward flow. Any increase in pressure in the right
ventricle may, sooner or later, cause heart failure. In some patients,
permanent structural changes may take place in the pulmonary arterioles,
producing very high right-sided pressures.

Symptoms and signs

About half the patients will have previously had at least one attack of rheumatic fever or rheumatic chorea. Typically, the patient is a young woman who has had no symptoms for many years but develops shortness of breath, at first only after severe exercise, but gradually after less and less exertion. Lying down may make her breathless and she may have to sleep propped up on pillows. Her sleep may be broken by attacks of breathlessness. She may suffer *haemoptysis* (coughing up blood), although this will usually not be severe. She may have particular trouble in pregnancy and, indeed, may develop acute pulmonary oedema and need an emergency operation, or even die. After child-bearing years, the breathlessness will continue and she may develop attacks of bronchitis each winter. Eventually atrial fibrillation will develop, paroxysmal at first, but eventually permanent. This will increase the breathlessness and may precipitate heart failure.

Atrial fibrillation encourages the formation of thrombus in the left atrium, already likely because of the stagnation of blood from the obstruction to flow. Emboli from such thrombus are common and may lead to a *hemiplegia* (paralysis of one side of the body) if cerebral, an acute abdominal catastrophe if mesenteric, or a gangrenous limb if femoral. Urgent surgery may be needed to save the patient. Mitral stenosis often presents as an embolus, often in a previously symptom-free patient.

Eventually, the patient will become more and more disabled. Blood will stagnate in peripheral veins, thrombus may form and pulmonary embolus and infarction result. Heart failure will respond to treatment for many years, but eventually death will occur. However, this course is often radically altered by surgical treatment.

On the other hand, many patients have milder stenosis and may lead a symptom-free normal life until they develop palpitations or heart failure from atrial fibrillation, at the age of perhaps eighty years.

The patient often has a characteristic facial expression (*mitral facies*) with cyanotic, dusky cheeks caused by long-standing poor flow through the skin blood vessels with resultant peripheral cyanosis. The pulse is of reduced volume and there is often atrial fibrillation.

In cases of advanced stenosis, the heave of the right ventricle under the sternum may be felt; the first heart sound (Figure 49) may be so loud

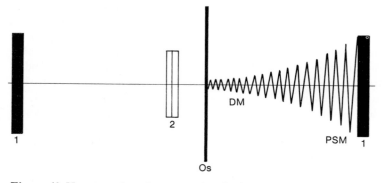

Figure 49 Heart sounds and murmurs in mitral stenosis.
D M represents a diastolic murmur and P S M a presystolic murmur

that it too can be felt. It may also be possible to feel a diastolic thrill. The second heart sound is usually normal, closely followed by a sharp sound called the *opening snap*. This is due to the movements of the cusps of the valve being suddenly stopped because they are stuck together. It is similar to the crack of a sail as it fills with wind, and is very characteristic of mitral stenosis. The snap is immediately followed by a diastolic murmur caused by the obstruction to the flow of blood through the valve which cannot open properly. At the end of diastole, the atrium contracts, blood is forced through the stenosed valve, and the murmur is increased in intensity (*pre-systolic murmur*) up to the loud first sound again. A systolic murmur may be heard as well, for the valve can neither close nor open properly, so some regurgitation may occur in systole. In atrial fibrillation the pre-systolic murmur will disappear. As the valve becomes calcified and less mobile, the first sound and opening snap get softer and the snap may disappear.

Diagnosis may be helped by the electrocardiogram, which shows the P waves of left atrial hypertrophy; the chest X-ray (Figure 50) may also help, showing the enlarged left atrium as well as evidence of engorged pulmonary veins and even pulmonary interstitial oedema at the bases. Calcium may also be seen on the valve during X-ray screening and the use of radio–opaque dye and cine-film will demonstrate the mobility and anatomy of the valve. Cardiac catheterization is seldom necessary but will show the pressure gradient from the left atrium to the left ventricle which indicates the severity of the stenosis. The size of the hole in the valve can be calculated from such measurements.

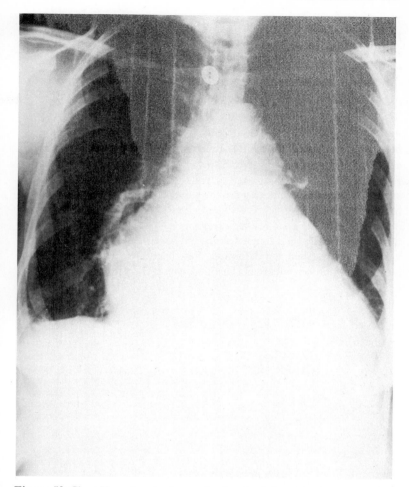

Figure 50 Chest X-ray in mitral stenosis, showing left atrial enlargement

A very useful investigation is to bounce ultrasonic sound waves off the anterior cusp of the mitral valve. This will show if the valve is stenosed, or if it is thickened, if calcification is present, and also the degree of mobility of the valve. This does not inconvenience or hurt the patient. All this information can help the surgeon decide what kind of operation is needed.

Treatment

If the patient is suffering from atrial fibrillation, digoxin must be used, although it is no use if the breathlessness is not caused by the rapid rate of fibrillation. There will also be the risk from emboli, so the patient should also be on anticoagulants, such as warfarin (Marevan). The patient usually attends a special anticoagulant clinic.

Surgical treatment is very valuable. Of the operations available, *closed mitral valvotomy* involves the introduction of a dilator through the beating left ventricle (Figure 51), directing it with a finger in the left atrium through the mitral valve. The dilator is then opened, splitting the fused edges of the cusps, and opening up the mitral valve orifice. In such cases, the surgeon cannot see the valve, but sometimes the valve is inspected and operated on directly (*open mitral valvotomy*). These operations produce good results, carry a very low risk and, if necessary, may be repeated several times. For patients over fifty years old, where the valve may be calcified and deformed, these operations may lead to severe mitral regurgitation and are not justified even if the patient has had an embolus.

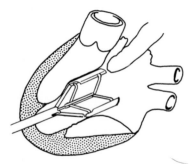

Figure 51 Transventricular mitral valvotomy

An alternative operation is to replace the mitral valve with a prosthetic valve, usually a Starr–Edwards valve, a ball in a cage (Figure 52). The mortality and morbidity is much higher in this operation than in mitral valvotomy at present, so it is considered only if the quality of the patient's life is very poor and he is likely to survive for only a very short time. However, surgical treatment is improving rapidly and patients not so seriously ill can now reasonably be considered for valve replacement.

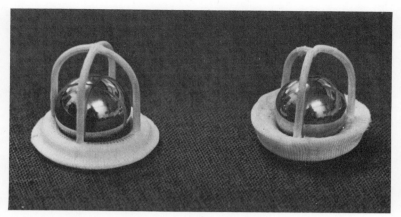

Figure 52 Starr–Edwards aortic and mitral valves.
The valve is a ball in a cage. The ball sinks to allow blood to pass through the valve, and then rises into its seating, preventing the blood from flowing back

Mitral regurgitation

When the mitral valve fails to close properly, some of the blood flows back into the left atrium, the chamber it has just left. This is known as regurgitation. This situation may occur on its own, or with mitral stenosis. There are six main causes:

1 *Rheumatic*, where the valve may be fibrosed and thickened with shortened chordae and a dilated mitral valve ring, so that the valve edges cannot meet and regurgitation of blood occurs.

2 *Subacute bacterial endocarditis* may destroy the valve tissue or rupture the cusps or chordae.

3 *Ischaemic heart disease* commonly causes minor degrees of regurgitation but myocardial infarction may involve the papillary muscle, allowing the cusps to balloon into the atrium and regurgitation to occur.

4 *Left ventricular failure* may cause the mitral ring to enlarge producing 'functional regurgitation' which often disappears on treatment.

5 *Congenital*, either alone or associated with other congenital abnormalities.

6 *Traumatic*, for example even non-penetrating injuries of the chest may sometimes cause the cusps, chordae or papillary muscles to rupture.

When mitral regurgitation occurs, the left atrium enlarges to accommodate the regurgitated blood. The pressures are not as great as those in mitral stenosis, so resultant severe pulmonary hypertension is less common. The left ventricle carries the added burden of the wasted output into the atrium, it dilates and may eventually fail. However, even severe regurgitation may be tolerated for many years. In sudden mitral regurgitation, for example when a cusp ruptures, the left atrium will be of normal size and will not dilate rapidly. This will lead to high pressure in the pulmonary veins and pulmonary oedema, and urgent operation may be needed.

Symptoms and signs
As with mitral stenosis, the patient may have suffered severe regurgitation for many years before symptoms occur, then some progress gradually and others very quickly. The chief symptoms are fatigue followed by breathlessness on effort, on lying down and paroxysmally at night. Atrial fibrillation increases the breathlessness. Like mitral stenosis, there is a tendency for embolism to occur and the risk of subacute bacterial endocarditis is greater. However, this usually occurs in mild rather than in severe regurgitation. Eventually, right-sided failure as well as left occurs.

The pulse is usually of small or normal volume and there may be atrial fibrillation. The apex beat is displaced to the left and has a sustained heaving impulse from the hypertrophied left ventricle. A systolic thrill may be felt. On auscultation (Figure 53), the first heart sound is soft and followed by a full-length systolic murmur. In early diastole, but after the opening snap position, a third heart sound is heard, often followed by a short diastolic murmur caused by the high flow from the over-distended left atrium through the mitral valve. The systolic murmur is heard round to the axilla.

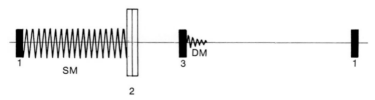

Figure 53 Sounds and murmurs of mitral regurgitation

The electrocardiogram may show evidence of an enlarged left atrium, if there is no atrial fibrillation and if the disease is severe, also a hypertrophied left ventricle (see p. 26). Chest X-rays will show evidence of left atrial and ventricular hypertrophy and, if the cause is rheumatic, calcification of the mitral valve may be seen. Angiography will show the degree of regurgitation, the size of the left atrium, the adequacy of ventricular contraction and the anatomy of the valve.

Treatment

Digoxin is used if the patient is suffering from atrial fibrillation, or if there is evidence of heart failure. If the patient is not expected to live long or if the quality of his life is poor, surgical treatment may be carried out, either to repair the valve or more usually to remove the diseased valve and suture in an artificial valve such as the Starr–Edwards valve. However, the risk is considerable and there are many complications, so the operation needs careful consideration and a clear understanding of the position by the patient. Where the patient has a mild degree of mitral regurgitation, it is essential to protect him against the possibility of subacute infective endocarditis. Thus, thirty minutes before any operation, however minor, such as dental scaling or extraction, he should be given 1 mega-unit of penicillin G and then penicillin V, 250 mg four times a day by mouth or sulphadimidine for three days afterwards.

The aortic valve

The aortic valve (Figure 54) is between the left ventricle and the aorta (see Figure 48). It consists of three cusps attached to a fibrous valve ring. Above the cusps are the dilatations of the aorta called the aortic sinuses (*sinuses of Valvsalva*). From the sinuses which correspond to the right and left cusps, the right and left coronary arteries arise. The third cusp is called the non-coronary cusp.

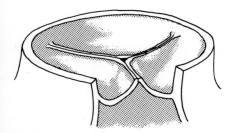

Figure 54 The aortic valve in the closed position

Aortic stenosis

In a number of people, there may be only two cusps to the aortic valve. It can thus never open fully and always obstructs blood flow to some extent. In later life, these valves tend to become calcified and stenosed and may lead to severe symptoms. Even normal valves may become involved in degenerative atherosclerotic changes and develop some stenosis. The rheumatic process may damage the cusps and lead to fibrosis and obstruction. There may also be some shrinkage of the cusps, giving aortic regurgitation as well.

Aortic stenosis may be rheumatic and usually then associated with mitral valve disease, atherosclerotic and then seldom severe, or congenital. Most cases of isolated aortic stenosis are congenital and most of these are of the valve itself, although occasionally stenosis occurs above or below the cusps which are then normal.

In severe stenosis, forward blood flow is impaired, and cardiac output reduced. The pressure difference across the valve may be as great as 100 mmHg, and the valve orifice may be little more than a pinhole. The left ventricle will hypertrophy to deal with the load, and maintain normal cardiac output for many years, but will eventually fail. The hypertrophied ventricle working excessively hard may make demands for oxygen that the coronary arteries cannot supply, and so cause anginal pain.

Symptoms and signs
Once symptoms of aortic stenosis have appeared, the outlook is poor and the patient is likely to die within a year or two. The early symptoms are fatigue, and breathlessness on exertion followed later by paroxysmal nocturnal breathlessness, and breathlessness on lying down (*orthopnoea*). Anginal pain is common and may be the result of excessive demands by the hypertrophied muscle and of associated ischaemic heart disease. Dizziness or loss of consciousness on exertion is very characteristic, and is ominous. It is probably caused by inadequate cerebral blood flow, resulting from a failure to increase cardiac output sufficiently during exercise, or by a transient abnormal rhythm. These patients are also liable to sudden death, often during exertion, presumably due to ventricular fibrillation or asystole.

Patients sometimes have a pale, delicate complexion ('Dresden china look'). If the stenosis is severe, the pulse is of small volume, rising slowly to its maximum. When taking the pulse with the finger, it feels as if it

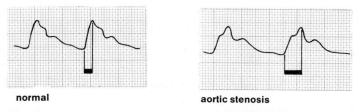

normal   **aortic stenosis**

Figure 55 Arterial pulse in aortic stenosis compared with normal

has a plateau (Figure 55). Atrial fibrillation would suggest that mitral valve disease is also present, since it is uncommon in aortic valve disease. The apex beat is often not displaced but is that of left ventricular hypertrophy, powerful and sustained. A systolic thrill may be felt at the base of the heart and in the neck. On auscultation (Figure 56) an atrial sound is heard. In early systole, the opening snap of the aortic valve, known as an *ejection click* is often heard. This is followed by a relatively short mid-systolic murmur that may also be heard in the neck. The second heart sound may be abnormal if the prolonged systole of the labouring left ventricle delays closure of the aortic valve. This means it is later than the pulmonary valve closure sound, and the splitting is therefore better heard in expiration than in inspiration. Often, however, it is not as bad as this and may appear to be single. The diseased aortic valve often makes little sound on closing and in a few cannot be heard at all.

The electrocardiogram shows marked left ventricular hypertrophy (see p. 26) if the stenosis is severe. X-rays may show left ventricular hypertrophy and calcification of the aortic valve. Cardiac catheterization will enable the pressure gradient across the valve to be measured. If surgery is contemplated, radio-opaque dye is injected into the coronary arteries

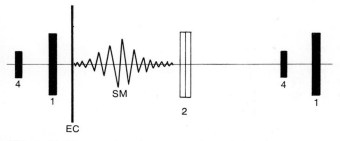

Figure 56 The sounds and murmurs of aortic stenosis.
4 represents the atrial (fourth) beat, while E C is the ejection click

and a cine-film X-ray is taken to assess whether or not there is any
disease in them, particularly if the patient has angina. Surgery for both
the valve and the coronary arteries, if diseased, is possible.

Treatment

If the disease is severe and it is possible to operate, surgical treatment is
usually carried out. The disease is said to be severe if the pressure gradient
across the valve is 60 mmHg or more, if there are symptoms referable to
the aortic stenosis, or if the electrocardiogram is worsening or the heart
is getting larger on X-ray. The age of the patient is not, in itself, a bar to
surgery – indeed most patients are elderly.

The operation is to remove the calcified diseased valve and to suture in
a Starr–Edwards valve, as large as the opening will permit. Alternatively
a *homograft* (Figure 57), a valve taken from a human heart at post-mortem
and specially prepared, or *heterograft*, a similar valve taken from a
non-human source such as a pig, may be used. Homografts are preferable
because they present no obstruction to the flow of blood, are quiet, and
do not require permanent anticoagulation. They may calcify in later years,
although some have been functioning well for up to ten years.

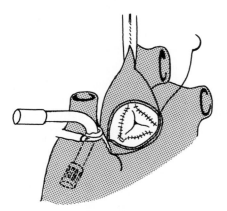

Figure 57 Aortic valve replacement – homograft

The complications of valve replacements are infection of the valve
(subacute infective endocarditis), haemolytic anaemia, due to damage to
the red blood cells as they hit the artificial valve, and embolism from
thrombus formation on the valve, which does not occur with homografts.

Those who survive and avoid the complications do very well indeed and usually go back to leading a normal life. It is an extremely satisfactory operation.

Aortic regurgitation

This is usually rheumatic and often associated with mitral valve disease. It may also occur in infective endocarditis when the valve is destroyed by the infection, in syphilis when the diseased ascending aorta dilates and may even become aneurysmal, and in dissecting aneurysm of the aorta when the medial coat is abnormally weak. It is occasionally congenital and may also occur in ankylosing spondylitis, rheumatoid arthritis and Reiter's disease. Sometimes an aortic cusp may rupture even without trauma to the chest wall.

In severe aortic regurgitation, a large volume of blood leaks back into the left ventricle in each diastole. If the ventricle is to propel a normal amount of blood into the aorta at each systole, it must dilate to accommodate the extra blood volume. Contraction will then be more powerful, but the ventricle will have to do more work and will eventually fail. Because of the large leak in diastole, the diastolic blood pressure will fall and the pulse pressure (systolic minus diastolic pressure) will increase.

Symptoms and signs
There may be no symptoms of aortic regurgitation for years but, when they appear, they are those of left ventricular failure, i.e. breathlessness on exertion, orthopnoea and paroxysmal nocturnal dyspnoea. Anginal pain is less common than with aortic stenosis.

These patients usually have a regular heart rhythm unless there is some associated mitral valve disease. Marked pulsation may be seen in the neck (*Corrigan's sign*) and the pulse is very characteristic, having a rapid rise and rapid fall (*collapsing pulse* or *water-hammer pulse*). The blood pressure tends to have a high systolic and low diastolic reading. The apex beat tends to be displaced and is very active because of the large volume so forcibly ejected at each heart beat.

A high-pitched, long diastolic murmur will be heard on auscultation, starting immediately after the second heart sound (aortic valve closure), and caused by the leak through the valve in diastole. There will also be a systolic murmur due to the excessive forward flow through the valve in systole (Figure 58). Sometimes the regurgitant flow of blood hits the anterior cusp of the mitral valve and causes it to vibrate. This may be

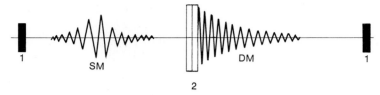

Figure 58 Sounds and murmurs of aortic regurgitation

heard as a rumbling low-pitched diastolic murmur at the base of the heart.

The electrocardiogram shows evidence of left ventricular hypertrophy (see p. 26) and X-rays show a large dilated left ventricle and a dilated descending aorta.

Treatment
In the earlier stages, much help can be obtained by the usual treatment for heart failure. If syphilis is the cause, it is treated with penicillin. As with aortic stenosis, the valve should be replaced if the disease is severe, but should not be left so long that the ventricular muscle has deteriorated beyond possible recovery. These patients often need combined medical and surgical treatment.

The tricuspid valve

The tricuspid valve is very similar to the mitral valve, except that it has three cusps. These cusps are controlled by two papillary muscles.

Tricuspid valve disease

Organic tricuspid valve disease is usually rheumatic, and there may be stenosis or regurgitation or both. Tricuspid regurgitation occurs in the congenital abnormality known as *Ebstein's disease* (see p. 141). Functional tricuspid regurgitation in right-sided heart failure from any cause is extremely common.

Tricuspid regurgitation

The symptoms are usually caused by the distension of the liver and by the other associated valve abnormalities present. If the cause is rheumatic, then other valves are also involved. The regurgitation of blood into the jugular veins produces a characteristic sustained surge in the neck, and this may be diagnostic. The liver is enlarged and may be seen and felt to pulsate. The right side of the heart is enlarged and the murmurs resemble those of mitral regurgitation, but are heard over the lower sternum and are often louder in inspiration as more blood flows into the right side of the heart. The electrocardiogram and X-rays (Figure 59) show right-sided heart enlargement, particularly of the right atrium.

If the regurgitation is functional, treatment of the heart failure often causes it to disappear. If it is organic, perhaps the result of rheumatic heart disease, then it may either be trivial and of no consequence or

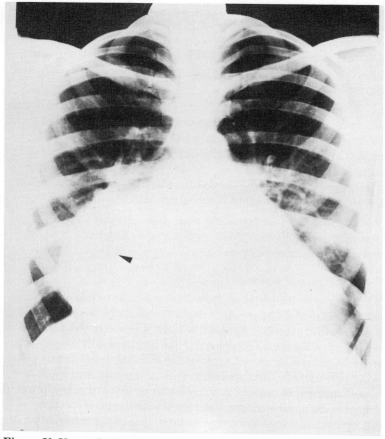

Figure 59 X-ray of tricuspid regurgitation.
Note the greatly enlarged right atrium (arrowed). The mitral and aortic valves are also diseased

severe, in which case repair of the valve or replacement with an artificial valve may be needed. Usually, if this is the case, the other valves will be badly diseased and will need to be replaced. It is possible to replace the mitral, aortic and the tricuspid valves in the same heart.

Tricuspid stenosis

The symptoms are mostly caused by the other valve lesions which are always present. Indeed, tricuspid stenosis may lead to less pulmonary congestion and less breathlessness. Sharp, flicking, 'a' waves may be seen in the veins of the neck as the powerful right atrium contracts against the stenosed tricuspid valve. However, if the rhythm is that of atrial fibrillation, this sign will not occur. The liver is enlarged and may pulsate in time with the venous 'a' wave. There may be ascites, and in heart disease this always suggests tricuspid valve disease or constrictive pericarditis.

In long-standing tricuspid stenosis, the patient may be jaundiced because of damage to the constantly distended liver (*cardiac cirrhosis*). The murmurs that may be heard are the same as those in mitral stenosis except that they have a tendency to increase in inspiration. Since mitral stenosis is usually present, it may be very difficult indeed to diagnose tricuspid stenosis clinically. However, cardiac catheterization will show a pressure gradient across the valve during diastole.

Tricuspid valvotomy is not usually carried out as it may lead to considerable regurgitation. Most cases can safely be left alone. Valve replacement is occasionally necessary.

Pulmonary valve disease

The anatomy of the pulmonary valve is very similar to that of the aortic valve. Disease of the pulmonary valve is almost always congenital, and is discussed on page 137. A rheumatic cause is very rare. Pulmonary regurgitation is usually functional and due to dilatation of the pulmonary artery, in pulmonary arterial hypertension from any cause. It may also occur after operation for pulmonary stenosis. It is suggested by an immediate diastolic murmur which is louder on inspiration and heard to the left of the upper sternum. However, it is sometimes difficult to differentiate from mild aortic regurgitation. Pulmonary regurgitation does not significantly affect blood flow through the heart and can usually be ignored.

Summary of nursing points

Certain events which occur in the cardiac cycle, such as the opening and closure of the valves which separate the chambers of the heart and those which separate the great vessels, the pulmonary artery and the aorta from the ventricles give rise to heart sounds. In disease of these valves, a disturbance of the sounds takes place and murmurs occur. The common conditions which lead to valvular disease are rheumatic fever and congenital heart disease. The nurse should observe the patient's temperature, pulse, blood pressure and respiration, and note and record any abnormality. She should observe the patient's colour and emotional state and also look for evidence of complications, such as infection, thrombosis and embolism.

The nursing management will depend on the severity of the condition but, in all cases, the nurse needs to be cheerful and to do everything possible to reassure the patient and enhance his morale.

The nurse should understand the principles of nursing care in such conditions as mitral stenosis and aortic stenosis. She should appreciate the clinical manifestations, pathology, investigations and treatment of these conditions. She should be able to prepare the patient for any investigations that may be necessary. She should also be aware of the pre- and post-operative care of the patient who is obliged to undergo corrective surgery, such as removal of a diseased valve and its replacement by means of a homograft or a Starr–Edwards valve.

Chapter 7

Congenital heart disease

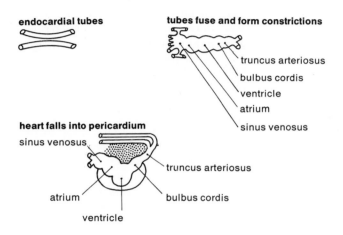

endocardial tubes

tubes fuse and form constrictions

truncus arteriosus

bulbus cordis

ventricle

atrium

sinus venosus

heart falls into pericardium

sinus venosus

truncus arteriosus

atrium

bulbus cordis

ventricle

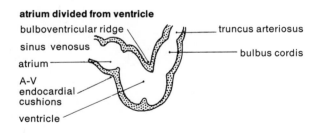

atrium divided from ventricle

bulboventricular ridge

sinus venosus

atrium

A-V endocardial cushions

ventricle

truncus arteriosus

bulbus cordis

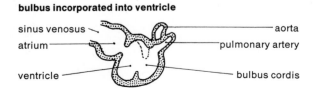

bulbus incorporated into ventricle

sinus venosus

atrium

ventricle

aorta

pulmonary artery

bulbus cordis

Figure 60 Early development of the heart.

Of all heart disease occurring in young patients up to fourteen years of age, 90 per cent is congenital. Eight out of every thousand live births have abnormal hearts, and in premature births the figure is as high as 24 per thousand. At present, about 80 per cent of these die within the first year of life. However, about 75 per cent of these babies can be helped so they will not die so soon, and may even live a long time. Many of them can be treated by palliative surgery, so that they survive to an age when further corrective surgery can be carried out. Many of those that will still die, will do so because they have multiple abnormalities which make life impossible.

Development of the heart

The heart develops from a straight tube which, in the first few weeks of embryonic life, twists into an S shape and divides into five parts by constrictions in the tube (Figure 60). These are:

the *sinus venosus*, into which the veins of the body drain
the *atrium*
the *ventricle*
the *bulbus cordis*
the *truncus arteriosus*.

The subsequent development may sometimes be abnormal and give rise to congenital heart disease.

Walls or *septa* appear and divide each atrial and ventricular chamber into two parts, as in the mature heart. The atria and ventricles are separated from each other by the growth of endocardial cushions; these also form the mitral and tricuspid valves. A spiral dividing septum is formed in the bulbus cordis and truncus arteriosus, leading to the formation of the outflow tracts of the ventricles, and into the aorta and pulmonary artery. After about two months of foetal life, the heart has more or less assumed its adult form.

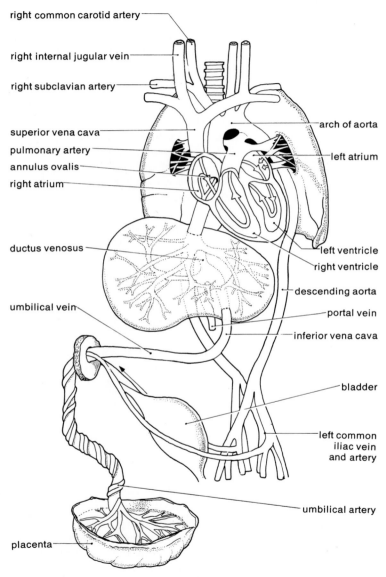

right common carotid artery

right internal jugular vein

right subclavian artery

superior vena cava

pulmonary artery

annulus ovalis

right atrium

arch of aorta

left atrium

ductus venosus

left ventricle

right ventricle

descending aorta

umbilical vein

portal vein

inferior vena cava

bladder

left common
iliac vein
and artery

umbilical artery

placenta

Figure 61 Foetal circulation

The blood circulating in the foetus (Figure 61) comes very close to that of the mother, in the placenta on the wall of the uterus. This allows the foetus to live and grow, as nutrients and gases dissolved in the blood pass across the thin endothelial membrane. The foetus receives oxygenated blood via the umbilical veins which lead from the placenta into the *ductus venosus* lying on the inferior surface of the liver. The ductus venosus is joined by the portal vein draining the gut, and then runs into the inferior vena cava bringing arterial blood to the right atrium. Only slight mixing occurs in the right atrium, most of the blood being diverted away from the right ventricle through the foramen ovale, which is open in the foetus, to the left atrium, left ventricle and aorta. The venous blood returns to the right atrium via the superior vena cava, and tends to flow through the tricuspid valve into the right ventricle and pulmonary artery.

The lungs need little blood because there is no foetal breathing. The lungs are not aerated and have a high resistance to blood flow, causing most of the blood to leave the pulmonary artery through the ductus arteriosus, thus reaching the descending aorta. This de-oxygenated blood eventually leaves the foetus by the two umbilical arteries arising from the internal iliac arteries and returns to the placenta, where it is oxygenated again. The pressures in the two ventricles of the foetal heart are the same and the right is as muscular a chamber as the left.

At birth, with the baby's first breath, the lungs become aerated and their resistance to blood flow decreases, so that more blood flows into them. At the same time, more blood flows back through the lungs to the pulmonary veins and left atrium, increasing the pressure and closing the flap-like foramen ovale to separate the two atrial chambers. The midwife ties the umbilical vessels, the ductus arteriosus closes, and the adult pattern of circulation is established. The physiological changes in the ductus arteriosus, ductus venosus, foramen ovale and umbilical vessels are sudden, but the anatomical changes are more gradual. It takes several months before these channels are obliterated, and even longer before the right ventricle becomes relatively much less thick than the left.

Diagnosis of heart failure in infants

Heart failure may appear very suddenly in infants, and indeed an inexperienced mother may not realize that anything is wrong. It is difficult to see raised jugular venous pressure in an infant, and there may be no peripheral oedema at first. There are, however, a number of features which a nurse may easily observe:

1 Failure to thrive may be associated with difficulty in feeding, with frequent pauses and lack of the strength to take the feed, and also with respiratory infections.

2 Sweating, possibly leading to a serious loss of sodium and potassium.

3 A rapid heart rate, which should not exceed 140 beats per minute during sleep in a healthy baby.

4 Rapid breathing.

5 Bulging of the chest wall due to over-distension of the lungs with blood.

6 Enlargement of the liver which can be felt.

7 Enlargement of the heart on the chest X-rays which, particularly in lateral views, may also show the lines caused by oedema of the lungs.

Some or all of these features may be found. There may be no murmurs to hear.

Central cyanosis would suggest the presence of congenital heart disease. This is caused by the shunting of blood from the right to the left side of the heart, or by inadequate blood flow through the lungs. Other possible causes of central cyanosis are: diaphragmatic hernia, diseases of the lungs, underventilation of the lungs or abnormal communications between the pulmonary and bronchial (systemic) arteries, called pulmonary arteriovenous fistulae. These can mostly be improved by the administration of oxygen, whereas the central cyanosis of congenital heart disease cannot. Clubbing of the fingers and toes may also occur, but usually not until the infant is from four to six weeks old. It is first seen in the thumb.

As well as the history, physical signs, electrocardiogram and radiographs, other important information for the diagnosis, which helps to plan the treatment, is obtained from cardiac catheterization.

Treatment of heart failure in infants

The treatment of all patients, whether they are adults, older children or infants is the same. But for the very young, there are certain additional points to be considered. These are:

1 Adequate sedation is needed.

2 Oxygen is essential and the aim should be to increase the oxygen content of the inspired air to 40 per cent.

3 Tube feeding is often necessary.

4 The patient may need to be nursed in a supportive frame or suspended in a propped-up position.

5 The body temperature in infants must be watched carefully, and overheating avoided, as the infant does not regulate its body temperature as well as an adult.

6 Infants will need relatively larger doses of digoxin than will older children. Digitilization can be obtained with a dose of digoxin of 70 μg/kg by mouth or 50 μg/kg intramuscularly. The daily maintainance dose is about 10 μg/kg (1 μg = 0·001 mg). For infants, digoxin can be made up in a paediatric mixture. For older children, Lanoxin PG, which contains digoxin 0·0625 mg (or 62·5 μg) in each tablet, is a useful preparation.

7 Diuretics are essential, but are likely to lead to potassium, calcium and magnesium depletion, so replacement of these may be necessary. Useful diuretics for infants are frusemide (Lasix) 1 mg/kg intramuscularly, mersalyl 0·2 ml intramuscularly or chlorothiazide 25 mg/kg by mouth.

8 Infections are often associated with heart failure and need energetic treatment.

9 Anaemia may also be present, and must be treated.

10 The cause of the heart failure should be diagnosed rapidly, because surgical treatment may be needed to save the life of some of these infants. They tolerate diagnostic procedures such as catheterization and even surgery remarkably well.

Diagnostic measurements and procedures
Cardiac catheterization

Fine catheters may be passed into the chambers of the heart, allowing samples to be taken and pressures to be measured (Figure 62). It is a simple technique seldom requiring anaesthesia (except perhaps for a fractious child), but sometimes requiring sedatives. The catheter is radio-opaque and can be guided to the required site using X-rays, with image intensification, displaying the picture on a television screen.

The right side of the heart can be catheterized by passing a catheter through a peripheral vein, usually the femoral or one in the elbow region. Samples can be taken and pressures measured in the superior and

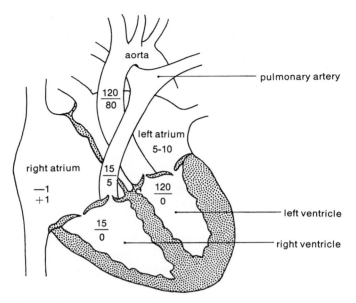

Figure 62 Pressures (in mmHg) in heart chambers and great vessels as measured at cardiac catheterization

inferior cavae, the right atrium, the right ventricle and the pulmonary arteries (Figure 63). By wedging the catheter into a pulmonary capillary, the 'wedge' pressure, which is a good indication of the left atrial pressure, can be recorded. In infants the catheter can be passed through the foramen ovale, enabling the left atrial and left ventricular pressures to be recorded directly. In older people, the inter-atrial septum may need to be punctured

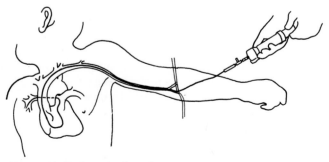

Figure 63 Catheter in the pulmonary artery

with a special catheter, in order to obtain access. Left-sided pressures and samples may also be obtained by passing the catheter up a peripheral artery, entered by a 'cut down' procedure or by a puncture technique.

The pressure waves are recorded on moving paper, with an electrocardiogram trace added to indicate the timing. Atrial pressure (see Figure 46) traces have two peaks and two troughs, labelled:

a corresponding to the contraction of the atrium

v corresponding to the contraction of the ventricle

x a descent corresponding to relaxation of the atrium

y a descent corresponding to the emptying of the atrium, as the tricuspid or mitral valve opens.

The a-wave will disappear in atrial fibrillation. It will be larger if there is high pressure in the pulmonary or systemic circulations, or if there is obstruction to flow from the atrioventricular valves onwards. High pressure y-waves may be seen in severe mitral or tricuspid regurgitation.

In infants, the pressures in the right side of the heart are high, taking some time to fall to the low adult levels. Normally the systemic arterial and ventricular systolic pressures are about six times as high on the left as on the right side. But in some congenital heart diseases, the right-sided pressures are very high indeed.

There is a notch on the descending limb of the arterial traces. This corresponds to the closing of the aortic and pulmonary valves. The subsequent pressure is the diastolic pressure.

Blood oxygen

A knowledge of the degree of saturation of samples of blood with oxygen is necessary for the measurement of blood flows, such as the cardiac output. Haemoglobin has a tremendous affinity for oxygen. Arterial blood normally contains 95 per cent of the amount of oxygen it could theoretically contain and is said to be 95 per cent saturated; when this is so, 1 litre is carrying 190 ml of oxygen. Venous blood is normally about 75 per cent saturated. The pressure of the oxygen in the plasma is the drive for this high level of saturation and is referred to as the oxygen·tension or pO_2. The air we breathe contains approximately 21 per cent oxygen so that the partial pressure of this will be about one fifth of normal atmospheric pressure ($\frac{1}{5} \times 760 = 152$ mmHg). In the alveoli of the lungs

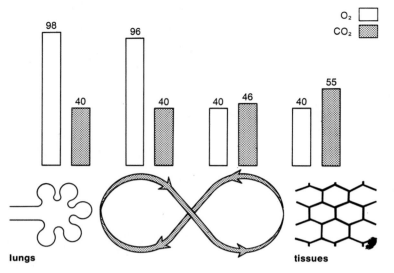

Figure 64 Partial pressures (mmHg) of oxygen and carbon dioxide in lungs and tissues

(Figure 64) it is rather less than this because part of the pressure is taken up by the pressure of water vapour which is present in these warm moist conditions and part by the pressure of carbon dioxide that is diffusing out of the blood. Thus, the partial pressure of oxygen is in fact about 100 mmHg. Since alveoli are not perfused with blood equally, there is a further small loss and the arterial oxygen tension tends to be about 90 mmHg.

Because of the great affinity of haemoglobin for oxygen, it is possible for this partial pressure to drop quite considerably before it has much effect on the oxygen saturation of the blood and, therefore, on the amount of oxygen carried and available. This means that one can climb to quite high altitudes and therefore lower partial pressures of oxygen and lower pO_2 levels in the blood before the oxygen saturation falls and symptoms occur. Venous blood has a pO_2 of about 40 mmHg.

It is also possible to measure pCO_2 (the tension or partial pressure of carbon dioxide) in the alveoli and blood (Figure 64). This may be a helpful measurement in differentiating the cyanosis of the respiratory distress syndrome (when it will be high) from that due to heart disease (when it will be normal).

Cardiac output

This is fundamental and is obtained by dividing the oxygen consumption by the lungs in one minute by the difference between the oxygen content in the pulmonary veins and that in the pulmonary artery:

$$\text{cardiac output (litres/min)} = \frac{\text{oxygen consumption (ml/min)}}{\text{arteriovenous oxygen difference (ml/litre)}}.$$

For example, if a normal adult extracts 250 ml of oxygen from the air he breathes in each minute, and the content of oxygen in samples from the pulmonary vein is 50 ml/litre greater than that in the pulmonary artery (*arteriovenous oxygen difference*), then 5 litres of blood must have passed through the lungs each minute (the cardiac output).

Pulmonary/systemic flow ratio

This helps decide the need for surgery in some conditions. Normally, the output of each ventricle is the same, but in some congenital heart disease, blood is shunted from left to right or from right to left, and outputs will not be the same. The pulmonary flow and the systemic flow have to be calculated separately. The pulmonary flow is calculated as in the example above, by dividing the oxygen consumption by the difference in the oxygen content in the pulmonary vein and that in the pulmonary artery. The systemic flow is obtained by dividing this same oxygen consumption by the difference in the oxygen content in the systemic veins (the right atrium is usually used) and that in a systemic artery, e.g. the femoral artery. From these two calculations, the ratio between the pulmonary flow and the systemic flow can be worked out.

Differences in the systemic and pulmonary blood flows indicate the occurrence of a shunt, usually from left to right and, less often, from right to left in congenital heart disease. Very small shunts and shunts in both directions are more difficult to detect in this way, and for them a special technique is used whereby a dye, such as *Cardio-green* or *Coomassie blue*, or other substances such as ascorbic acid or radioactive gas, is injected into the heart chambers or great vessels, and the time it takes to reach other parts of the heart or great vessels is measured by picking up the injected substance with a photoelectric cell, or by other means. A shunt can be detected by measuring the time between the first appearance of the dye and its reappearance after having circulated again. The cardiac output can be calculated by drawing a graph of the changing concentrations of the dye in the circulating blood.

Vascular resistance

A knowledge of this can also help in deciding the advisability of surgical treatment. Pulmonary and systemic resistance to flow can be calculated using Poiseuilles' equation:

$$\text{resistance} = \frac{\text{pressure gradient}}{\text{flow}}.$$

The pulmonary and systemic flows have been calculated as shown above. The pulmonary gradient is the difference in the pressures (in mmHg) in the pulmonary artery and in the left atrium; the systemic gradient is the difference between the pressures in the aorta and in the right atrium. Since pressures change throughout the cardiac cycle, a mean or average pressure is used. Thus, the pulmonary resistance is found by dividing the pulmonary pressure gradient by the pulmonary flow, and similarly for the systemic resistance. Resistance is usually recorded in simple units. In the foetus, as described above, the pulmonary resistance is high and this state may persist or may return in later life. This may lead to high right-sided pressures causing shunting of blood from right to left with resultant central cyanosis.

Congenital heart disease

Little is known of the causes of congenital heart disease. Perhaps the best known cause is the german measles (*rubella*) virus. If the mother catches rubella in the first three months of pregnancy, there is a considerable chance that the child will be born with a persistent ductus arteriosus or pulmonary stenosis, and the child may also have nerve deafness, cataracts and be mentally defective (Figure 65). This risk is considered so great that termination of the pregnancy is usually advised. If gamma globulin is given within a few days of exposure to this infection, it may be prevented. It is possible that other viruses may be similarly harmful.

The notorious drug *thalidomide* not only left a legacy of limb abnormalities, but also of congenital heart defects. Indeed, as few drugs as possible should be taken during pregnancy for others, too, may be risky. Exposure to radiation is also harmful.

Congenital heart disease may be associated with other congenital abnormalities. For example, in *Down's syndrome* (mongolism), the children have 47 chromosomes instead of the normal 46. The extra one is an additional 21-chromosome and the disorder is called *21 trisomy*.

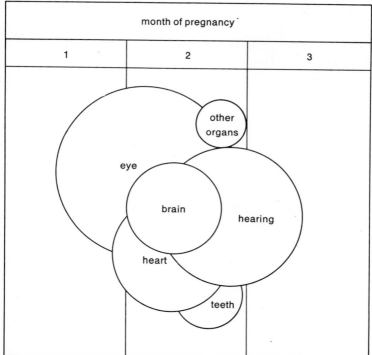

Figure 65 The effects of German measles during pregnancy

Twenty per cent of children with Down's syndrome have ventricular or atrial septal defects.

In any family where one member is known to have a congenital heart abnormality, there is an increased likelihood of other members having abnormal hearts, although it is unusual for identical twins to both have congenital heart disease. If one child in a family is affected, the risk of the second being affected is 1 in 25. If two children are affected, the risk to the third is 1 in 12. However, the kind of abnormality is also important, for some can be relatively easily corrected, while others are impossible to correct and will lead to invalidism and to a shortened life.

Congenital heart disease is classified in various ways, such as into *cyanotic* and *non-cyanotic* or into those with *left-to-right shunts*, those with *right-to-left shunts* and those with *no shunts* or into those with *communications between*

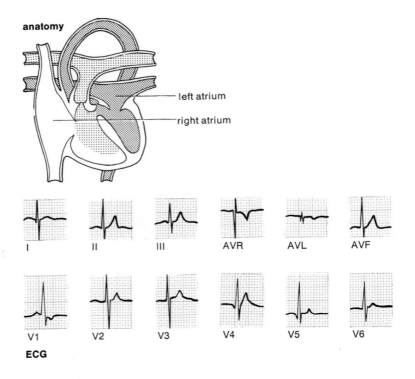

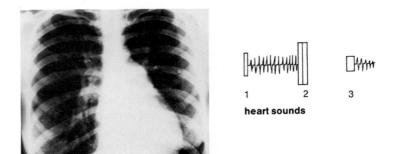

X-ray

Figure 66 Ventricular septal defect

the systemic (left) and pulmonary (right) circulations, those with *obstructive lesions* (e.g. valve stenosis) and those with *displacement of heart chambers, vessels or valves*.

No classification is really satisfactory and, indeed, multiple abnormalities which defy simple classification are common. Some of the more common and important congenital heart defects will now be described.

Ventricular septal defect

This is the most common form of congenital heart disease (Figure 66). A large number, perhaps as many as a third, close spontaneously. If this is going to happen it will have done so by about ten years of age. The ventricular septum is made up partly of membrane and partly of muscle, and holes (sometimes more than one) may occur in either part, but are most commonly found in the membranous septum below the tricuspid valve. Blood will usually be shunted from the left (high pressure) side to the right (low pressure) side.

If the defect is small, the main risk will be from subacute infective endocarditis. If the defect is large, the flow of blood through the right side may be several times the systemic flow, and severe heart failure may develop. This is particularly liable to occur as the high vascular resistance in the lungs of the foetus gradually falls to allow a bigger shunt; so heart failure is common at the age of two to three months. If no symptoms occur while the patient is young, he may live for many years without trouble. But, in some, breathlessness or fatigue may herald the beginning of heart failure in later life.

There are three main physical signs of the condition:

1 There may be evidence of left and right ventricular enlargement.

2 A long systolic thrill may be felt and a long systolic murmur heard close to the lower left sternal edge.

3 If the defect is large a third heart sound may be heard at the apex, together with a short diastolic murmur due to the high blood flow through the mitral valve.

In small defects, the electrocardiogram will be normal, but in large ones, there may be evidence of hypertrophy of both ventricles. The chest X-ray will be normal in small defects, but in large ones will show enlargement of the heart and prominent pulmonary blood vessels due to the overfilled lungs. Cardiac catheterization will allow the size of the shunt to be calculated, and X-ray pictures taken after the injection of radio-opaque dye will show the position of the defect.

Small defects need no treatment, although penicillin must be given before dental treatment and operations to avoid subacute infective endocarditis. Large defects should be closed but, because of the high mortality rate if this is done in infancy, it should be delayed until later in life. If heart failure occurs in infancy, a palliative procedure such as tying a ligature around the pulmonary artery (*banding*) should be carried out to reduce the pulmonary blood flow.

Atrial septal defect

There are two types of atrial septal defect, those occurring away from the atrioventricular valves (*ostium secundum*) and, less common, those occurring near them (*ostium primum*). The latter are caused by faulty formation of the endocardial cushions which separate the atria from the ventricles as well as the fault in the septum which separates the left and right atria. The endocardial cushion defect may lead to mitral and tricuspid regurgitation, because the valve leaflets are involved in the developmental failure. A ventricular septal defect may be present as well. Sometimes there is an associated abnormality when some or all of the four pulmonary veins drain into the right instead of into the left atrium.

With an atrial septal defect (Figure 67), the atria tend to behave as in a single chamber. Because the right ventricle is a thinner structure with a lower pressure, the right side of the heart becomes filled preferentially, and there may be an increase in pulmonary blood flow of 2 or 3 times the systemic flow. However, this is tolerated well, and symptoms do not usually appear until middle life, when atrial dysrhythmias such as flutter or fibrillation occur, eventually followed by congestive cardiac failure. Occasionally no symptoms appear until much later in life.

The physical signs are not striking, so the diagnosis is often missed. There may be evidence of right ventricular hypertrophy. The second heart sound is widely split and does not vary with respiration. This is because the increase in heart filling during inspiration is shared equally by both atria, and so pulmonary and aortic valve closure remains a constant time apart, the pulmonary valve closing later because of the much larger volume of blood being handled by the right side. There is usually a systolic murmur caused by high blood flow through the pulmonary valve, and there may be a diastolic murmur due to high blood

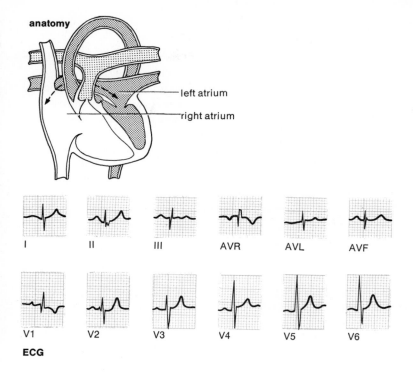

anatomy

— left atrium
— right atrium

I II III AVR AVL AVF

V1 V2 V3 V4 V5 V6

ECG

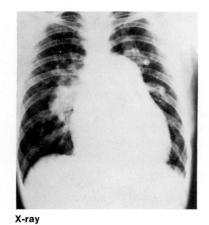

1 2 3
heart sounds

X-ray
Figure 67 Atrial septal defect

flow through the tricuspid valve. In primum defects, the long murmurs of mitral and tricuspid regurgitation may be heard.

The electrocardiogram nearly always shows right bundle branch block. This may be complete, but is usually partial, with splintering of the QRS complex in lead V1. In the rarer ostium primum defect, the axis is leftward instead of rightward or normal. The X-ray usually shows some heart enlargement and conspicuously large pulmonary arteries, which when seen by X-ray screening pulsate vigorously. This is known as the *hilar dance*. Catheterization allows the size of the shunt to be calculated, and may show the presence of abnormal drainage of pulmonary veins into the right atrium. In a primum defect, mitral regurgitation may be demonstrated by passing a catheter through the defect into the left atrium and left ventricle, and then injecting radio-opaque dye.

A secundum defect may be closed with very little risk, and this is usually recommended if the pulmonary flow is more than twice the systemic flow. Correction of a primum defect, with its associated valve clefts, is much more risky, and is usually undertaken only if there are incapacitating symptoms or if the shunt is very large.

Persistent ductus arteriosus

Normally, the ductus arteriosus narrows and closes within a few days of an infant's birth; sometimes, however, it remains open. If this happens, blood flows continuously from the high-pressure aorta to the low-pressure pulmonary artery. If the flow is very large, it will lead to heart failure in the first few weeks of life, and urgent surgery may be needed. Usually there are no symptoms, the characteristic murmur being heard later in life.

If the shunt is large, a characteristic pulse, known as a *collapsing pulse* may be felt. There is an abrupt pulse rise felt and a sudden subsidence. The diastolic blood pressure will be low, and there may be evidence of left ventricular hypertrophy. The most characteristic sign is a continuous murmur heard over the ductus in the second left intercostal space close to the sternum (Figure 68). In a large duct, there may also be a murmur due to high mitral diastolic flow from the greatly increased amount of blood returned from the lungs to the left atrium.

The electrocardiogram is usually normal, but may show left ventricular hypertrophy (see p. 26). The chest X-ray may show some enlargement of

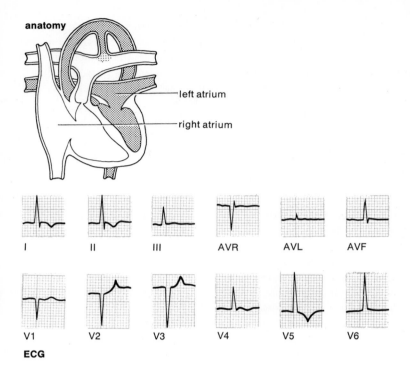

anatomy

left atrium

right atrium

I II III AVR AVL AVF

V1 V2 V3 V4 V5 V6

ECG

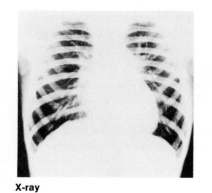

X-ray

1 2

heart sounds

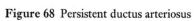

Figure 68 Persistent ductus arteriosus

the left side of the heart and an increase in the blood vessel markings in the lungs due to the large pulmonary blood flow. Catheterization is seldom necessary, but it is possible to pass the catheter from the pulmonary artery through the ductus arteriosus into the descending aorta. The duct may also be shown up by angiography using radio-opaque dye.

Surgical closure of the ductus, by ligation or division between sutures, carries a very low mortality, and should usually be done before the child starts school. If it is not done, there is a risk of subacute infective endocarditis and of left ventricular failure in later life.

The Eisenmenger syndrome

Eisenmenger described a 'complex' in which there was a right-to-left shunt with central cyanosis and clubbing in ventricular septal defect, even in the absence of pulmonary stenosis. More recently, this 'complex' has been enlarged into a syndrome embracing all those conditions in which, without pulmonary stenosis, central cyanosis is caused by a shunt from right to left. This is less common than a shunt from left to right, and is brought about by an increase in resistance in the pulmonary circulation leading to a considerable rise in the right-sided pressures. This brings them above the left-sided ones, thus causing the shunt to change from left-to-right to right-to-left. This can be caused by a persistence of the high foetal pulmonary vascular resistance and so present from birth, or it can be due to an acquired high pulmonary vascular resistance as a reaction to long and persistently high pulmonary flow. The most common connections between the left and right circulations to 'react' like this are ventricular and atrial septal defects and persistent ductus arteriosus. For reasons that are not understood, if this is to happen it is most common from birth in ventricular septal defect and persistent ductus arteriosus, but in later life in atrial septal defect. When the shunt is reversed in this manner, the patient becomes cyanosed and clubbing occurs.

The characteristic physical signs of the congenital abnormality tend to disappear and are replaced by those of pulmonary arterial hypertension. There will be evidence of right ventricular hypertrophy, a dominant 'a' wave in the jugular pulse, a pulmonary ejection click and systolic murmur, loud pulmonary valve closure and often the murmur of pulmonary regurgitation (Figure 69).

It may be difficult to recognize the underlying cause. In ventricular septal defect, the pressures in the two ventricles are equal, so the pulmonary and

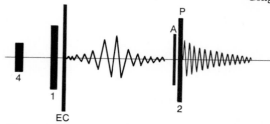

Figure 69 Heart sounds and murmurs of pulmonary arterial hypertension in the Eisenmenger syndrome

aortic valves will close at the same time giving a single second sound; in persistent ductus arteriosus, the split of the second sound will widen during inspiration as occurs normally; and in atrial septal defect the second sound will remain widely split with no variation with respiration. Patients may complain of breathlessness, angina from the poor cardiac output, loss of consciousness on exertion because they cannot adequately increase cardiac output and haemoptysis. They will eventually develop congestive cardiac failure.

The situation is a perilous one, yet many live into adult life. The defect cannot be corrected because of the high pulmonary vascular resistance. The right-to-left shunt is a safety valve and, if it is stopped, right-sided heart failure will ensue, and the patient will die. The only possible treatment would be transplantation of the lungs and heart together, but this is not yet possible. Pregnancy is exceptionally hazardous and must be avoided. The contraceptive pill often leads to pulmonary thrombosis and increase of the pulmonary vascular resistance, so this must be avoided as well. Sterilization is justifiable.

Fallot's tetralogy

This is the most common cause of cyanotic congenital heart disease in children surviving infancy (Figure 70). The four features of the tetralogy are:

1 Severe pulmonary stenosis. This may be of the valve itself, of the infundibulum in the part of the right ventricle leading up to the valve, or both.

2 A large ventricular septal defect.

3 Overriding of the origin of the aorta astride the ventricular septal defect.

4 Hypertrophy of the right ventricle.

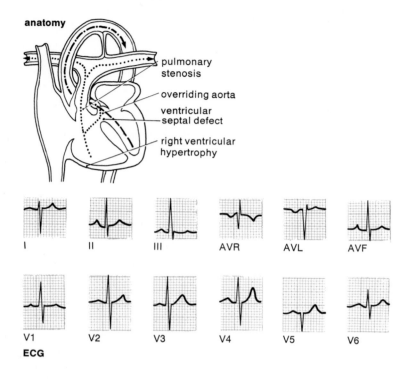

anatomy

pulmonary stenosis

overriding aorta

ventricular septal defect

right ventricular hypertrophy

I II III AVR AVL AVF

V1 V2 V3 V4 V5 V6

ECG

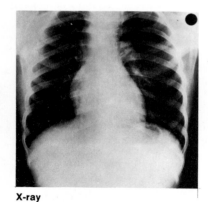

X-ray

heart sounds

Figure 70 Fallot's tetralogy

Because of the severe stenosis of the normal outlet from the right ventricle, the pressure in the right ventricle rises to the same level as that in the left, and blood is shunted from right to left, producing central cyanosis. In very severe cases the cyanosis may be present from birth, but usually it appears later in childhood and gradually worsens as the infundibulum of the right ventricle gets progressively narrower. These children may get sudden cyanotic attacks with much deeper cyanosis and indeed they may look black and even lose consciousness. As the cyanosis gets worse they get more breathless. A very characteristic feature is squatting (Figure 71); the child spontaneously learns to squat after exertion. This possibly decreases the shunt by increasing the resistance in the large arteries of the legs and abdomen.

On examination, the child may be poorly developed. There will be central cyanosis and clubbing of the fingers and toes. A loud systolic murmur and thrill from the pulmonary outflow tract will be heard, and the second heart sound will be single because the diseased pulmonary valve closes so softly that it is inaudible (Figure 70).

The electrocardiogram will show evidence of right ventricular hypertrophy. The chest X-ray characteristically shows a boot-shaped heart; the toe is formed by the small left ventricle lifted up on the large right ventricle, and the instep is the concavity, resulting from the poorly developed pulmonary artery beyond the severe stenosis.

In an endeavour to overcome the anoxia, more red cells are produced (*polycythaemia*), so the haemoglobin level is high and the packed-cell volume increased.

Diagnosis at the bedside is usually not difficult. Cardiac catheterization will demonstrate equal pressures in the right and left ventricles, the pressure gradient across the pulmonary valve indicating the severity of the lesion and the degree of oxygen desaturation in the aorta. The injection of radio-opaque dye will demonstrate the anatomy, and is of great importance in considering surgical treatment.

Usually untreated children with this disease die in childhood, although an occasional patient may survive to middle age. Death may be from a cyanotic attack, from cerebral abscess (to which they are prone), from cerebral thrombosis because of the increased viscosity of their polycythaemic blood, or from infective endocarditis.

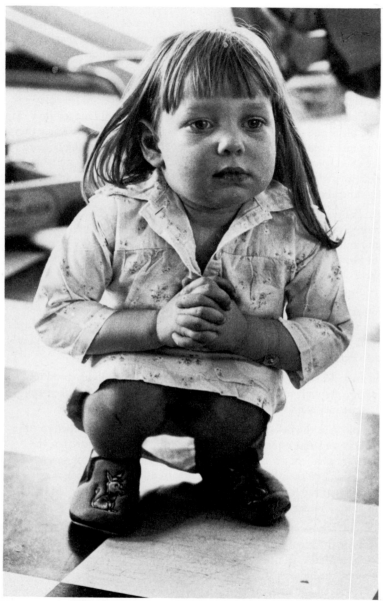

Figure 71 Child squatting in position typical of Fallot's tetralogy

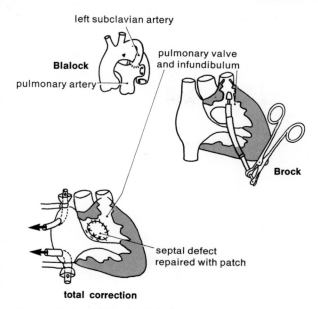

Figure 72 Operations for Fallot's tetralogy

Surgical treatment (Figure 72) is usually necessary. If an infant is severely ill, it may be necessary to carry out a quick palliative operation in the hope that a proper corrective operation may be done at a later age. In the *Blalock operation*, the right or left subclavian artery is anastomosed to the pulmonary artery. This increases the amount of blood flowing to the lungs to be oxygenated. The *Brock operation* is to open up the stenosed pulmonary valve and to punch out some of the infundibulum to relieve the stenosis, and thereby increase the flow to the lungs. This will also decrease the right-sided pressure and the right-to-left shunt. Although these procedures carry a high mortality in infancy, they still frequently save life. In older children, it is often possible to do a corrective operation in one stage, patching the ventricular septal defect and opening up the pulmonary valve and infundibulum.

Pulmonary stenosis

This is a common disorder (Figure 73) and is usually congenital. Stenosis of the valve itself is usually seen alone, but stenosis in the infundibular region is often associated with other abnormalities. The severity may vary

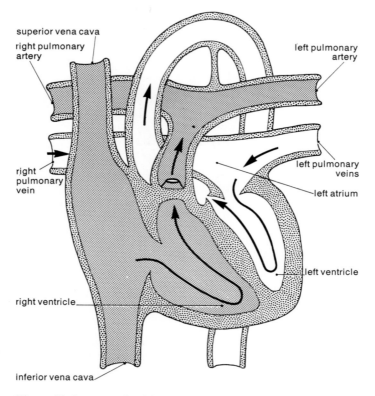

Figure 73 Anatomy of pulmonary stenosis

enormously from an unimportant lesion to almost total blockage of the valve. It is usually discovered during routine examination but, if it is very severe, it may cause congestive heart failure early in life. Loss of consciousness on exertion may occur owing to the inadequate blood supply to the brain, the heart being unable to increase its output.

If the stenosis is severe, a prominent 'a' wave may be seen in the jugular pulse as the right atrium contracts against the hypertrophied right ventricle. There will be evidence of right ventricular hypertrophy and, in the second left intercostal space close to the sternum, a thrill will be felt, and the characteristic short systolic murmur heard following a click (the *ejection click*) caused by the opening of the abnormal valve. Because of the difficulty and the increased time of emptying the blood from the right ventricle through the stenosed valve, the pulmonary valve will close late and the second heart sound will be widely split. The actual sound of the pulmonary valve closing will be soft or, if very severe, inaudible. The electrocardiogram will show varying degrees of right ventricular hypertrophy depending on the severity, and in mild cases it will be normal. In severe cases the chest X-ray will show absolutely clear lung fields, because of the poor pulmonary blood flow caused by the extreme obstruction, and the characteristic dilatation of the main pulmonary artery beyond the obstruction. Catheterization will enable the pressure gradient across the valve to be measured, and thus the degree of obstruction can be calculated. In very severe cases, the pressure in the right ventricle may be much higher than that in the left ventricle. When the catheter is drawn back through the valve from the pulmonary artery to the right ventricle, a sudden change of pressure can be seen, as the stenosed valve is crossed. It is thus possible to determine whether the stenosis is at the level of the valve, the infundibulum or both.

In severe or moderately severe cases, the narrowed valve is usually opened up surgically.

Coarctation of the aorta

In this abnormality, the aorta is severely narrowed, usually just beyond the origin of the left subclavian artery. It may be associated with an abnormal aortic valve which has two instead of three cusps, and has become stenosed or regurgitant. Hardly any blood flows through the narrow part of the aorta, so the circulation to the lower part of the body is accomplished by the enlargement of what are normally small arteries and the opening up of anastomotic channels to bypass the narrow segment. These may be seen and felt clinically, particularly around the scapular regions.

The enlarged intercostal arteries produce characteristic notches on the underside of the ribs which can be seen in the chest X-ray. The femoral pulses are of diminished volume, and there is a delay in the arrival of the pulse wave when it is timed against the carotid pulse. The blood pressure in the lower limbs is low, but raised in the upper limbs. A systolic murmur may be heard over the coarctation. In most patients there are no symptoms, but heart failure may occur in infancy.

The diagnosis is usually made in later life, being brought to light by the heart murmur, hypertension or a complication. The high blood pressure may eventually lead to left ventricular failure, and the coarcted area or a bicuspid aortic valve is liable to bacterial infection. In some patients, there is an abnormal aorta and this may rupture or tear on the inside and allow blood to track along between the layers of the aortic wall (*dissecting aneurysm*, see p. 181). These patients may also have small aneurysms on other arteries, particularly those in the brain, and they may die from rupture of one of these (*subarachnoid haemorrhage*).

Diagnosis is not difficult, but X-rays using radio-opaque dyes may demonstrate the anatomy accurately before surgery, which is nearly always advisable whether there are symptoms or not. The affected part of the aorta is resected and the ends joined by anastomosis; if this is impossible a Dacron graft is inserted.

Transposition of the great arteries

This occurs when the septum that divides the bulbus cordis and truncus arteriosus develops in a straight line, instead of in the usual spiral manner. There are several types, but in the most important, the aorta arises from the right ventricle and the pulmonary artery from the left ventricle (Figure 74). The pulmonary and systemic circulations are then entirely separate, and life is impossible. In those who survive, there is a communication between the two sides achieved by a persistent foramen ovale, an atrial septal defect, a ventricular septal defect or a persistent ductus arteriosus. The infant is usually cyanosed from birth, has feeding difficulties, goes into heart failure and dies within a few weeks. Physical signs are not very helpful. This defect is the most common cause of cyanosis and heart failure in the first few days of life, and urgent investigation is essential. Catheterization and angiography will show that the aorta arises from the right ventricle, and lies in front of the pulmonary artery instead of behind it, as would be normal. A recent exciting discovery is that these infants can be treated at the time of catheterization. The operation is the *balloon septostomy*: a special catheter is passed from the right atrium through the foramen ovale (usually easy in the infant) into the left atrium, the balloon is inflated and pulled briskly back through the foramen ovale, tearing the septum to produce an atrial septal defect. This procedure is repeated until the hole is large enough to allow considerable flow of blood in each direction. This usually leads to improvement and the infant survives long enough for later corrective surgery.

Later on, in early childhood, the atrial septum is removed and patches of pericardium inserted to divert the pulmonary vein blood to the aorta and caval blood to the pulmonary artery, albeit still via the wrong ventricle.

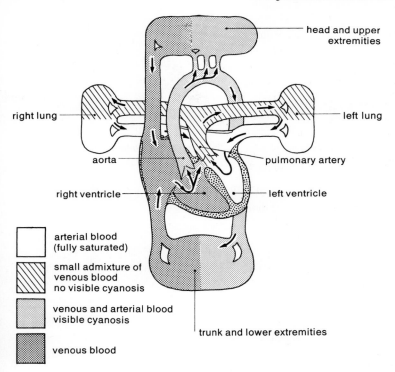

head and upper extremities

right lung

left lung

aorta

pulmonary artery

right ventricle

left ventricle

☐ arterial blood
(fully saturated)

◩ small admixture of
venous blood
no visible cyanosis

▦ venous and arterial blood
visible cyanosis

▨ venous blood

trunk and lower extremities

Figure 74 Transposition of the great arteries

Other congenital heart abnormalities

Some less common abnormalities are listed below:

Aortic stenosis
This (see p. 106) is usually seen in later life when a bicuspid (instead of tricuspid) valve becomes calcified and stenosed.

Ebstein's anomaly
The tricuspid valve is displaced downwards into the right ventricle, and there is tricuspid regurgitation. An atrial septal defect is usually also present.

Dextrocardia
In this, the heart is a mirror image of its usual self (Figure 75). This is often associated with mirror image inversion of all the other organs of

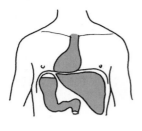 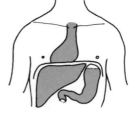

situs inversus   **isolated dextrocardia**

Figure 75 Types of dextrocardia

the body (situs inversus). If it is not then the heart is usually abnormal, with multiple congenital defects.

Double outlet right ventricle
This occurs when both the aorta and the pulmonary artery arise from the right ventricle. A ventricular septal defect allows blood to flow between the left and right sides.

Pulmonary atresia
The outflow tract from the right ventricle fails to develop. The pulmonary circulation is thus dependent on the bronchial arteries and veins which, because they are enlarged, cause a continuous murmur over the lungs.

Persistent truncus arteriosus
The spiral septum completely fails to develop, so that only one great vessel arises from the heart with only one valve at its origin, sitting astride a ventricular septal defect, collecting blood from both left and right ventricles.

Tricuspid atresia
The tricuspid valve fails to develop. For survival there must be an atrial septal defect together with either a ventricular septal defect or a persistent ductus arteriosus, to obtain a pulmonary circulation.

Anomalous pulmonary venous drainage
There are various types of this disorder. The pulmonary veins drain into the right atrium instead of the left. If all four do, an atrial septal defect is necessary for survival.

Cor triatriatum

This is a heart with three atria. In fact, a membrane with a perforation in it divides the left atrium into two compartments. Clinically it looks like mitral stenosis.

Heart surgery

Surgical operation for congenital heart disease may be palliative or corrective. The common palliative procedures are designed either to reduce or increase pulmonary blood flow, or to increase the mixing between the two circulations.

Pulmonary blood flow may be reduced by tying a ligature around (*banding*) a pulmonary artery, e.g. in a large ventricular defect in infancy when far too much blood reaches the lungs.

Pulmonary blood flow may be increased and central cyanosis relieved in two main ways:

1 By decreasing the obstruction, e.g. opening up a stenosed pulmonary valve and infundibulum as in Brock's operation for Fallot's tetralogy.

2 By creating an artificial shunt between the pulmonary and systemic circulations. This may be done in three places: (a) between a subclavian artery and a pulmonary artery (the *Blalock operation*), (b) between the descending thoracic aorta and the left pulmonary artery (the *Potts operation*), (c) between the ascending aorta and the right pulmonary artery (the *Waterston operation*).

Increasing mixing between the two circulations used to involve the creation of a large atrial septal defect, as in the Blalock–Hanlon operation used in treating transposition of the great arteries. This carried a high mortality and a procedure known as a *balloon septostomy* was devised by Rashkind in which a special catheter with a balloon on the end is passed from the right atrium through the foramen ovale, which is usually easy in an infant, into the left atrium. The balloon is then inflated and pulled briskly back through the foramen ovale, tearing the septum to produce an atrial septal defect.

As well as these palliative operations, many congenital heart defects can be partially or totally corrected. An accurate diagnosis is essential and the patient should be well prepared; heart failure and any lung infections should have been treated, and any anaemia or electrolyte imbalance corrected. Heart surgery may be closed or open. In *closed heart surgery*,

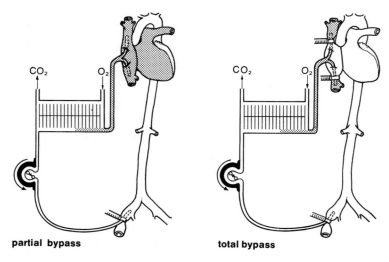

partial bypass   **total bypass**

Figure 76 Cardiopulmonary bypass

the heart continues to circulate blood. This is used in the shunt operations described above, and in operations for persistent ductus arteriosus, coarction of the aorta and the Brock operation for pulmonary stenosis. In *open heart surgery*, the heart and lungs are excluded from the circulation, their functions being taken over by a pump and an artificial oxygenator.

The venous blood is taken by tubes inserted into the superior and inferior vena cavae to the oxygenator, and is then pumped back into the circulation through a tube into a femoral artery. All or part (*total* or *partial* bypass) of the blood may be dealt with in this way (Figure 76).

In a total bypass, the heart will be dry except for blood returned by the coronary circulation through the coronary sinus to the right atrium, and some blood from the bronchial circulation returned by the pulmonary veins to the left atrium. This blood can be sucked out, and pumped through a defoamer back to the oxygenator. When the aortic valve is being operated on, it is also necessary to cannulate the two coronary arteries, and feed them with blood from the oxygenator.

There are several different types of oxygenator. *Bubble* oxygenators bubble oxygen through the blood and then defoam it with silicone. *Stationary screen* and *rotating disc* oxygenators bring a thin film of blood into contact with oxygen on a still screen or rotating disc. Membrane oxygenators, like the lung, have a thin membrane between the blood and the oxygen

However, essential though they are, oxygenators tend to damage the blood. The use of a membrane protects the red cells and other blood constituents. Better 'breathing' membranes are currently being developed.

Post-operative care

There are four main points which are important in post-operative care:

1 The tissues must be kept oxygenated. Therefore, humidified oxygen is given and secretions are cleared by suction. Encouraging breathing and physiotherapy also help. Sometimes positive pressure ventilation may be necessary.

2 The acid–base balance should be carefully watched. Low cardiac output and poor tissue perfusion together with inadequate respiratory function may lead to tissue anoxia, and the accumulation of lactic acid. This can be corrected by giving sodium bicarbonate intravenously.

3 The normal blood volume must be maintained. Blood loss, as it occurs at operation, must be replaced, and the fluid intake and output subsequently adjusted, to allow for hidden fluid loss such as by respiration and sweating.

4 A careful watch must be kept for complications such as heart failure, tamponade from bleeding into the pericardium, haemothorax, pulmonary embolism, dysrhythmias, respiratory failure such as *perfusion lung* (patchy areas of collapse through which blood still flows but which cannot be oxygenated, thereby lowering the arterial oxygen saturation), renal failure and cerebral damage from anoxia, emboli or oedema.

Summary of nursing points

To understand congenital heart disease, the nurse must understand the way in which the heart develops, together with its general anatomy. She should appreciate the high rate of incidence of congenital heart abnormalities in order to grasp the magnitude of the problem.

The nurse should understand such conditions as atrial septal defect, ventricular septal defect, persistent ductus arteriosis and Fallot's tetralogy. She must be conversant with the principles of investigation and treatment in these conditions.

As the patients affected are usually children, additional problems of nursing management are involved. These relate to the physical, emotional and social care of the patient. The nurse must do everything to minimize emotional trauma to the patient and enhance his uneventful recovery.

Chapter 8   The lungs and pulmonary circulation in heart disease

The lungs receive blood from the heart, oxygenate it, remove carbon dioxide and then return it to the heart, from where it is pumped into the systemic circulation. Chronic disease of the lungs may thus affect the heart in various ways.

The pulmonary circulation

The outflow tract of the right ventricle of the heart pumps blood through the *pulmonary valve* into the main *pulmonary artery* (Figure 77). This artery immediately divides into two main branches, the right and the left. The short systolic murmur commonly heard in healthy people is due to the turbulence of the blood at the branching point. The right and

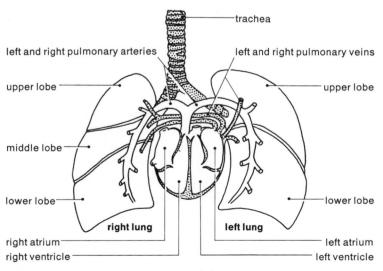

Figure 77 Diagram of pulmonary circulation

left pulmonary arteries then divide further to supply the lobes of the two lungs. More subdivisions occur until the terminal capillaries reach the alveoli, where they anastomose with the pulmonary vein and bronchial artery capillaries.

The pressures in the pulmonary circulation are about one-sixth of those in the systemic circulation – the pulmonary artery pressure is about 20/10 mmHg. The flow at the base of the lung is nine times as much as that at the top of the lung, owing to the effect of gravity. This forms a useful reserve in case of any extra demand, for example, during exercise or to compensate for the effects of some diseases, since it allows a considerable increase in the amount of blood flow without any increase in the pulmonary artery pressure. Pulmonary arteries and arterioles have layers of muscle in their walls which are under nervous control, so they may dilate or constrict, varying the *pulmonary vascular resistance*, in order to control the flow. This resistance can be measured using a cardiac catheter (see p. 124). When the resistance is increased, the pressure in the pulmonary arteries will increase resulting in right ventricular hypertrophy and eventually even right-sided failure.

The main function of the pulmonary circulation is to allow the exchange of oxygen and carbon dioxide between the air in the alveoli and the blood. The capillaries are so small that the blood is spread out into a very thin layer and is only separated from the air in the alveoli by a layer of endothelial cells. This means there is very good contact between the blood and the air: oxygen passes one way and dissolves in the blood, and carbon dioxide in the blood passes across in the opposite direction and mixes with the air. This exchange occurs rapidly and efficiently. The process cannot take place, of course, if there is any obstruction present. For example, in pulmonary oedema, there is a thin layer of fluid in the walls of the alveoli, and this seriously interferes with the exchange process.

Acute pulmonary embolism

Thrombi are always being formed in the veins and small *emboli* (blood clots) often find their way into the lungs. However, they do not cause much damage because the lung has two alternative blood supplies, pulmonary and bronchial, which can keep it alive while the embolus is destroyed by enzymes. Thus the lung acts as a good filter. However, if large thrombi form, and large emboli pass from the veins through the right side of the heart to the pulmonary arteries, they may block the outflow of the right ventricle, either at the pulmonary valve or at the point where the main pulmonary artery divides. This will completely obstruct the circulation and result in rapid death. Alternatively, they may move on and block a large pulmonary artery, and obstruct that, or they may break up and reach the smaller vessels. If the bronchial circulation beyond the obstruction cannot adequately supply the tissues with blood, they will die (*pulmonary infarction*) and pleurisy may occur over the infarcted area, showing itself as pleuritic pain, a pleural rub and a pleural effusion. The embolus usually comes from the leg or pelvic veins, although it may come from the right side of the heart, in cardiomyopathies, for example.

Patients with heart disease are more likely to have a sluggish blood circulation and to produce emboli. If their lungs are congested, they may have difficulty in dealing with the emboli. Anyone confined to bed is at some risk from this disorder, so as few patients as possible should be allowed to remain in bed. There is also a risk of the blood clotting after a coronary thrombosis, after an operation and after childbirth, particularly if the patient is kept long in bed. Recently, more pulmonary emboli have been found in young people, often without any obvious cause. There may be a minor trauma, or a leg in plaster; women taking contraceptive pills run a greater risk. Some diseases, such as polycythaemia and malignant disease, can also be complicated by thrombus formation.

There can be a large amount of clot in the leg veins of patients in bed, with no clinical evidence of it. To prevent this potential danger, the patient should be encouraged to get up out of bed as soon as possible or, if this is not possible, to do frequent leg exercises, say for five minutes in each hour. Early signs of deep venous thrombosis to watch for are: pain in the leg, swelling of one leg, discoloration of the skin and tenderness along a clotted superficial vein. Thrombus formation in veins is very dangerous, there is always more thrombus than suspected, so early treatment with anticoagulant drugs is essential. Recent work suggests that small doses of *heparin* given subcutaneously may prevent the formation of blood clot.

Symptoms and signs

It is important to recognize the slightest hint of a pulmonary embolus at the earliest possible moment. Small emboli often herald major emboli which might be prevented. There may be no symptoms at all or, even with a large embolus, merely slight chest pain, slight haemoptysis, unexplained rapid breathing or rapid heart rate. However, the obstruction to the circulation may cause the patient to collapse and lose consciousness, or he may suffer severe chest pain, indistinguishable from that of myocardial infarction, and due to poor coronary blood flow. The pleuritic pain of infarction occurs later and is not nearly so ominous a symptom. Proper anticoagulant treatment at an early stage may well prevent later death from a massive embolism.

If the embolus is small, the patient may look well, but if it is massive, he will appear pale, cold and sweaty, with cyanosis of the extremities. The blood pressure and pulse volume will be low, the heart rate fast, and the jugular venous pressure may be raised. A right-sided atrial sound may usually be heard and, occasionally, systolic and diastolic murmurs may be heard if there is an embolus in a large pulmonary artery.

Deep venous thrombosis in a leg may make it reddened, oedematous and tender, or there may be only a little oedema, a tender superficial vein or calf tenderness on stretching the Achilles tendon (*Homan's sign*).

Unfortunately, it is common for there to be complete blockage of deep veins with no physical signs at all, but this can be diagnosed using an ultrasonic technique or more accurately by venography (injecting radio-opaque dye into the veins of the legs).

The electrocardiogram may be very helpful, a typical pattern being shown in Figure 78. However, many varieties occur. There may be right axis deviation, partial or complete right bundle branch block, tall peaked P waves, T wave inversion from V2 to V4, or atrial dysrhythmias. These changes may be transient, so they may not always be seen and their absence does not disprove the diagnosis. Even in massive embolism, the X-ray may be normal. However, it may show linear scars from previous smaller emboli, or a picture similar to that of pulmonary oedema. The right diaphragm may be raised and later a pleural effusion may be seen or a wedge-shaped shadow of pulmonary infarction. Pulmonary angiography, with radio-opaque dye, will show the blockage of the pulmonary arteries and the poor filling of the blood vessels beyond them. A useful technique

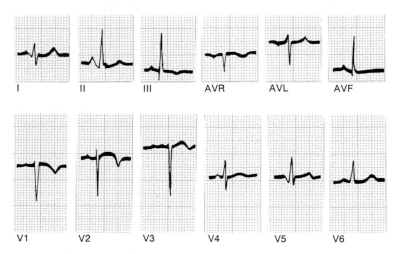

Figure 78 Electrocardiogram of acute pulmonary embolism

is to inject albumin labelled with radioactive iodine and then to 'scan' the lung, to show the areas with poor blood perfusion.

Treatment

Patients should be nursed in the most comfortable position and given 6 to 8 litres of oxygen per minute by mask or by double nasal catheter. Anticoagulants are the most important part of treatment, and should be started immediately, whether the episode is a minor or a major one. Heparin should be given by continuous intravenous infusion controlled by clotting times measured at the bedside or by the cephalin–kaolin time measured in the laboratory. Usually, about 40 000 units are needed in each 24 hours, and the effects are often dramatic. This treatment should be continued for ten to fourteen days, and then replaced by oral anticoagulants such as warfarin, whose dosage is controlled by the prothrombin time. This anticoagulant regime is continued for six months. Fibrinolytic substances such as streptokinase and urokinase help to dissolve the emboli and to return the pulmonary circulation to normal, but they are exceedingly expensive. Pain may be relieved with pethidine but never with morphine as this may depress the respiratory centre. Digoxin may be needed if atrial fibrillation occurs, or together with diuretics if there is heart failure as well. The patient will either die at once (10 per cent) or within a few hours (a further 20 per cent) or respond rapidly to treatment and make a complete recovery. Occasionally, a patient remains with an obstructed pulmonary circulation and hypotension, and surgical removal of the embolus might then be attempted, using a cardiopulmonary bypass technique, but the survival rate is disappointingly low.

Prevention

This is extremely important. We have already seen the value of getting patients out of bed as soon as possible or, if this is not possible, instituting leg exercises. If the patient is confined to bed, elastic stockings may help and so may a simple apparatus which rhythmically compresses the calves and keeps venous blood moving. Anticoagulant drugs may be used in some susceptible patients, such as those with a myocardial infarction. Even small doses of heparin given subcutaneously have been shown to be useful prophylactically after operations. Operative treatment has been tried such as tying off the inferior vena cava or lessening flow through it by taking a tuck in it (*plicating*). But, collateral venous channels soon grow and they will allow emboli to pass. Clots in the peripheral veins can be removed in an operation using Fogarty's venous catheter.

Pulmonary arterial hypertension

Hypertension in the pulmonary circulation is just as important as hypertension in the systemic circulation. It is different from pulmonary venous hypertension, which is a back pressure resulting from the rise in pressure in the left atrium usually due to mitral stenosis or left ventricular failure, and which may lead to pulmonary oedema. The upper limit of pressure in the pulmonary arteries is no more than 30/15. It may be raised in several ways:

1 From increased pulmonary blood flow. This may occur when there is a large shunt of blood from left to right, as in septal defects and persistent ductus arteriosus. At first the little-used pulmonary vessels are dilated to accommodate more blood, with no rise in pressure. However, when the pulmonary flow becomes as large as three times the systemic flow, increases of pressure in the pulmonary arteries are needed to maintain the circulation.

2 Following on increased pulmonary capillary pressure (*pulmonary venous hypertension*). This follows an increase in the left atrial pressure and therefore the capillary pressure that occurs in mitral stenosis and left ventricular failure. It is initially not severe, but may eventually increase

pulmonary vascular resistance, with permanent changes in the structure of the small pulmonary vessels, and lead to considerable rises of pressure.

3 From increased pulmonary vascular resistance. This may be due to constriction of the pulmonary arterioles as a reaction to low oxygen tension in the blood (*hypoxia*) or to persistently raised capillary pressure. It is particularly common in mitral stenosis but may occur in left ventricular failure. Effective surgery in mitral stenosis may reverse it.

4 The pulmonary arterioles may also become constricted by disease with a thickening of the muscular coat (*media*) and an increased resistance to blood flow. This may have been present from birth or it may have been acquired. It may be seen in congenital heart disease with communications between the left and right sides (the Eisenmenger syndrome, see p. 132). Pulmonary arteriolar changes may also result from long-standing pulmonary hypertension due to any cause.

5 The small arterioles may be obstructed, perhaps by emboli, and then secondary changes take place in their elastic and muscular coats making the obstruction permanent. After childbirth, repeated small emboli from pelvic or leg veins may give rise to permanent pulmonary arterial hypertension. A very severe variety is seen in the tropics, the embolus being the eggs of an infesting worm (*Schistosoma mansoni, haematobium* or *japonica*).

Combinations of these causes often occur.

Symptoms and signs
The characteristic symptoms are fatigue and breathlessness on exertion. In severe cases, there may be anginal pain because obstructed flow in the pulmonary circulation lowers cardiac output and, therefore, coronary flow. The low output may also affect the cerebral circulation and cause unconsciousness or dizziness on exertion. Haemoptysis may occur. Eventually, there will be right-sided heart failure with oedema.

The signs, whatever the cause, are characteristic. The pulse volume is low. A prominent 'a' wave may be seen in the jugular pulse in the neck due to the powerful right atrial contraction. The heave of right ventricular hypertrophy may be seen and felt. There may be a pulmonary ejection click and a systolic murmur over the dilated pulmonary artery, as well as a right-sided atrial sound. The pulmonary valve is slammed shut loudly and early by the high diastolic pressure, so the second heart sound will be unusually narrowly split and will sound abnormally loud. The pulmonary valve may allow regurgitation and produce a diastolic murmur. Later, heart failure may occur with its characteristic signs.

The electrocardiogram shows the pattern of right ventricular and right atrial hypertrophy (see p. 31). Chest X-rays show large main pulmonary arteries and abnormally clear lung fields because of poor perfusion of blood through them.

Treatment
This depends on the cause. Many patients go on for years before heart failure occurs. If there is evidence that the cause is recurrent emboli from the venous circulation, permanent anticoagulant treatment will be necessary. However, the more usual patient with a large pulmonary embolus will either die, or make a good recovery with no permanent damage. Permanent and severe pulmonary arterial hypertension occurs only with the recurrent small emboli usually presenting as dyspnoea in a young woman after childbirth.

Pulmonary heart disease (cor pulmonale)

This is a form of pulmonary arterial hypertension caused by disease of the respiratory system which has secondary effects on the heart. It is very common, although it is becoming less so as a result of efforts to keep the air clean. Chronic bronchitis worsened by air pollution, cold, damp winters and cigarette smoking is much the most common cause.

The low tension of oxygen in the alveoli in the lungs leads to constriction of the arterioles. The walls of the alveoli rupture, so there is a loss of perfusion surface. The small pulmonary blood vessels are obliterated by fibrosis and thrombus, and the capillaries are compressed when air is trapped in the alveoli causing a high intra-alveolar pressure. These mechanisms lead to an increase in pulmonary vascular resistance which causes an increase in right-sided pressures in the heart, and then right ventricular hypertrophy and, eventually, right-sided heart failure. The work of the right ventricle is further increased by *polycythaemia*. This is an increase in the number of red blood cells. It may help transport more oxygen for a time but also increases the viscosity (stickiness) of the blood, so the heart has to work harder to force it round the circulation. The poor oxygenation of the tissues generally also affects the myocardium.

There are many causes of pulmonary heart disease. *Chronic bronchitis* is extremely common and often leads to it. *Emphysema* is also common, and may not be associated with chronic bronchitis. In both cases there is a tendency for air to be trapped in the alveoli and for some alveoli either to be uselessly perfused because they are poorly ventilated or for them to be uselessly ventilated because they are poorly perfused. *Bronchial asthma* can also cause pulmonary heart disease, but not as often as chronic bronchitis and emphysema. Tuberculosis, industrial dust hazards, bronchiectasis, irradiation given for carcinoma of the lung or breast, and diffuse interstitial fibrosis may all lead to pulmonary heart disease. Thoracic deformities such as severe kyphoscoliosis and the old operation for tuberculosis, *thoracoplasty*, may also cause it. Difficulties in breathing leading to inadequately ventilated lungs, for example, after poliomyelitis, or from the mechanical difficulty due to extreme obesity may cause pulmonary heart disease. In a few people there is an inadequate central drive from the brain to breathe, and these people therefore ventilate inadequately and may get pulmonary heart disease. There are also many other less important causes.

Symptoms and signs

The patient is often breathless and wheezing, and may or may not be cyanosed. If carbon dioxide has accumulated in his blood, it may lead to mental confusion and trembling hands. The hands tend to be warm and the pulses bounding because the blood vessels at the periphery are dilated, and there may be clubbing of the fingers. There may be evidence of heart failure. The failing right heart often enlarges, the tricuspid ring distends and marked tricuspid regurgitation results giving a large venous pulse in the neck and a large pulsatile liver. The chest may be barrel-shaped and may move very poorly on respiration. Breath sounds may be poor and added rhonchi and crepitations may be heard. It is often difficult, because of the lung disease, to detect the signs of right heart enlargement and pulmonary hypertension. A third heart sound may be heard if there is heart failure and the murmur of tricuspid regurgitation may also be heard, although this can be severe without a murmur being heard.

The X-ray changes depend upon the nature of the causative disease and there may even be none. The electrocardiogram may be normal or may show the typical P wave of right atrial hypertrophy and evidence of right ventricular hypertrophy or right bundle branch block (see p. 31). It may only become abnormal at the time of additional infection.

Pulmonary function tests and blood gas estimations will be abnormal, and they may help decide the nature of the underlying lung disease. Carbon dioxide in excess in the blood (raised pCO_2) almost always means that there is some pulmonary contribution to heart failure.

Treatment
Oxygen is the first essential and is given with a special mask (Figure 79), delivering 28 per cent oxygen. If too much oxygen is given, respiration may decrease and carbon dioxide retention occur, leading to mental confusion or coma. This is because a low oxygen tension has become the stimulant to the respiratory centre in the brain instead of the normal stimulant of a high carbon dioxide tension. If a mask is not adequate, it may be necessary to use intermittent positive pressure respiration achieved with a mechanical ventilator and tracheal intubation or tracheostomy.

Infection will always be present in these irreparably damaged lungs, so wide-spectrum antibiotics should be given. Suitable ones are ampicillin, or oxytetracycline in doses of 250–500 mg every six hours, for as long as necessary. Spasm may be overcome by bronchial dilators and such drugs

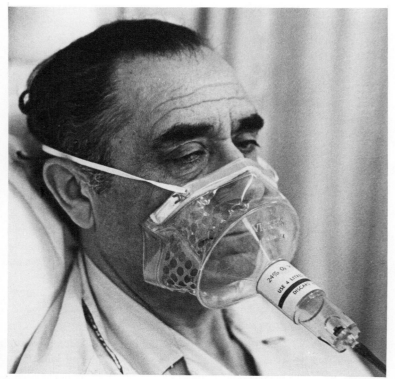

Figure 79 Oxygen mask

as intravenous aminophylline, 500 mg, isoprenaline in 10–20 mg doses by mouth or salbutamol or orciprenaline by inhaler are used. In severe asthma, steroids such as prednisone by mouth, hydrocortisone or ACTH by injection may be useful and even save life. Digoxin and diuretics are used in the usual way to treat congestive heart failure. Sedatives all tend to depress respiration and should be avoided if possible. Morphine is particularly dangerous and should never be used. If there is severe polycythaemia – packed cell volume (PCV) over 55 per cent – the viscosity can be reduced by taking off some blood and replacing it with *rheomacrodex*, which has the same molecular weight as normal blood.

Prevention
Smoking cigarettes must be stopped, and dusty, cold, damp, foggy atmospheres avoided. Any respiratory infections should be treated at once, and some patients need to be kept on antibiotics throughout each winter. Many of these patients, cardiac and respiratory cripples, will die in a severe attack. However, if they recover and efforts are made to prevent recurrences, some may continue for a long while to lead a reasonable and fairly comfortable life.

Summary of nursing points

The nurse should appreciate the relevance of the pulmonary circulation in physiology as a whole. She should also understand the importance of the anatomical relationship between the heart and the lungs, as this knowledge is vital in appreciating the significance of any pathological condition that may result. There are three main conditions which may occur: acute pulmonary embolism, pulmonary arterial hypertension and pulmonary heart disease.

The nurse must understand the principles of nursing care and management of the patient with any of these conditions. Where a patient is being given an anticoagulant drug, the nurse must observe all orifices for signs of haemorrhage. She must also ensure, by constant vigilance and advice to the patient, that no contra-indicated item of diet is given. When oxygen is being given, the nurse must ensure that all precautions are taken to prevent accident, and that the oxygen is given as prescribed. She must be alert for signs of oxygen intoxication.

The more detailed form of nursing management must include observation of the patient's temperature, pulse, respiration rate and blood pressure, together with fluid balance, diet, cough, degree of breathlessness and emotional reaction. The prescribed treatment in respect of rest, diet and drugs must be carried out scrupulously. If the patient is on complete bed rest, everything must be done for him, including feeding and bathing. Care of the skin is vital, as frequently the tissues are oedematous and are liable to abrasion and infection. Regular turning of the patient should be effected; and, if necessary, the patient may be nursed on a ripple bed. The nurse should be capable of preparing for any procedures (investigations) that may be performed by the doctor.

Chapter 9

Pericardial, myocardial and endocardial disease

The heart is composed of three structures, the *pericardium*, the *myocardium* and the *endocardium*. The pericardium is the membrane surrounding the heart, the myocardium is the heart muscle, and the endocardium lines the myocardium and also forms the valves.

The pericardium

This is the thin membranous sac completely surrounding the heart. It is composed of simple epithelial, squamous and cuboidal cells, and an underlying layer of fibro-elastic connective tissue. Although thin, it is strong and prevents overdistension of the heart in diastole. However, if it is removed, this does not seem to lead to any trouble.

Acute pericarditis

This is acute inflammation of the pericardium. There are many causes, perhaps the most common is that following *myocardial infarction*. The common, so-called idiopathic benign variety may be caused by a virus. The virus is usually *Coxsackie B*, but occasionally it may be influenza virus or some other type. It is not always benign, for it may be recurrent and may lead to *constrictive pericarditis*. Pericarditis may occur in rheumatic fever or as a result of damage due to bacterial infection, when the sac will contain pus. It is common in severe uraemia. It occurs in collagen disorders such as rheumatoid arthritis, polyarteritis nodosa and systemic lupus erythematosus. It may be tuberculous and in some tropical areas this is the most common variety. It may be due to invading malignant disease such as carcinoma of the lung. It may also result from injury or surgery to the heart or nearby structures.

Symptoms and signs
Acute pericarditis is often heralded by sudden chest pain, usually in the centre of the chest but sometimes in the shoulders, arms or back. It is

similar to the pain of myocardial infarction, but tends to vary with respiration, position and swallowing. The patient may feel less pain if he sits up or leans forward. The pain may last for weeks. There may be a preceding respiratory infection in the viral variety.

The doctor may have to make the diagnosis on the history alone. However, a sound known as a *pericardial friction rub* may be heard with a stethoscope. This is a curious scratching sound, often having systolic and diastolic elements, but not quite in time with the heart sounds. It may vary with respiration, and it may be fleeting or transitory, so frequent examinations may be necessary. The patient should be sitting up and leaning forward.

The electrocardiogram (Figure 80) is often helpful, although it may be normal. Frequent serial records should be taken. Usually, all the leads show raised S T segments with an upward concavity differing from those of myocardial infarction. As the disease progresses, the S T segments come down and the T waves become inverted.

A chest X-ray is not usually helpful unless a pericardial effusion occurs. It is often said that the serum enzymes (S G O T, for example) are not

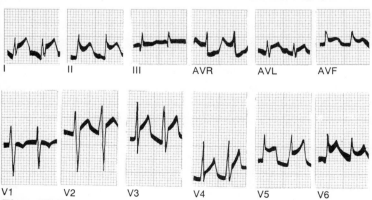

Figure 80 Electrocardiogram of acute pericarditis

raised in pericarditis, thus distinguishing it from acute myocardial infarction. Unfortunately, this is not so. A moderate rise is common and not surprising, since some of the muscle underlying the pericardium is always damaged.

Diagnosis

In *viral pericarditis*, the virus may be found in the faeces, or occasionally in the blood or pericardial fluid. It may be possible to show a rising level of antibody to the virus obtained by examining two blood samples taken at ten-day intervals. *Bacterial pericarditis* usually causes a great deal of toxicity and there is usually a pericardial effusion which is purulent and from which the bacterial organism can be grown. *Tuberculous pericarditis* also causes an effusion, and this may contain blood and excess protein. The tubercle bacillus can usually be grown from the fluid. Other causes will have the characteristic features of the generalized disease concerned.

Pericardial effusion

This can occur in any kind of pericarditis. It may also occur in heart failure, owing to simple *transudation* (passing out through the membranes) of fluid, but here it is of little consequence. If the effusion is large, a very dull percussion note may be heard over the heart area when the chest is percussed, and the heart sounds may be faint. However, it is most frequently noticed on a chest X-ray, the heart shadow being large and globular in shape (Figure 81). If the action of the heart is observed on an X-ray screen, little pulsation will be seen. The diagnosis is proved by removing some fluid through a needle. The fluid may be examined for cells, protein and organisms. At the time the fluid is taken off, air or carbon dioxide may be injected into the pericardial sac, and X-rays will then show whether the pericardium is thick, as may be the case with tuberculous pericarditis. This can be important, as an early operation may be desirable. Pericardial effusion can also be demonstrated by passing a cardiac catheter into the right atrium against its lateral wall, when X-rays will show up any fluid or thickened pericardium. A valuable new diagnostic technique involves bouncing ultrasonic sound waves off the heart, when two echoes will be recorded instead of the normal one.

Pericardial tamponade

This is caused by a rise in pressure inside the pericardial sac (Figure 82). This rise obstructs normal ventricular filling and eventually leads to a poor

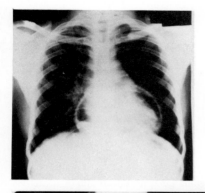

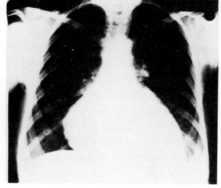

Figure 81 Pericardial effusion and pericardial thickening shown by injecting air into the pericardial sac

cardiac output and death if not treated. When the ventricles cannot dilate properly in diastole, the pressures go up and, as a result, the pressures in the systemic and pulmonary veins increase. Stroke output is low, so a rapid heart rate occurs to compensate for this. Pressure in the jugular veins will be high and so-called *arterial pulsus paradoxus* occurs. In the normal person, blood is held back in the lungs during inspiration, and left-sided output decreases. This may be detected by a diminished pulse volume in inspiration. In pericardial tamponade, this is much accentuated and, if found in quiet respiration, provides a valuable physical sign.

Treatment
The patient with acute pericarditis should be nursed in the most comfortable position. The pain may necessitate analgesics in the early

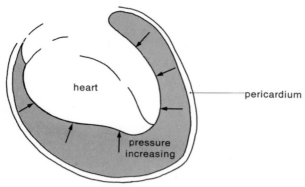

Figure 82 Pericardial tamponade – bleeding into the pericardium gradually compresses the heart

stages. Tuberculosis will need treatment with anti-tuberculous drugs, and bacterial infections with antibiotics and, often, the removal of the pus. The virus infections subside spontaneously, but recurrent attacks may occur. If they are prolonged or recurrent or tamponade occurs, steroids such as *prednisone* are valuable. If myocardial infarction is the cause, anticoagulants must be stopped because of the risk of bleeding into the pericardial sac. This may cause tamponade (Figure 82). Whatever the cause of tamponade, urgent drainage of the pericardial sac may be necessary. Prednisone is also used in the treatment of collagen disorders.

Chronic constrictive pericarditis

In this condition, the pericardium becomes thickened, and may become fibrosed and calcified, particularly if the cause is tuberculosis. Strands of diseased tissue may extend into the myocardium beneath and damage it. The heart is then constricted and unable to fill properly. The condition may often have no obvious cause. It may sometimes follow rheumatoid arthritis, or be due to viral pericarditis or tuberculosis. (Tuberculosis is the most usual cause of the condition in underdeveloped countries.) In rare cases, it may be caused by irradiation to the chest, or by invasion from cancer or following purulent pericarditis.

Chronic constrictive pericarditis is remediable, but it may be misdiagnosed. For example, the patient may be thought to be suffering from congestive cardiac failure, and may even have had an abdominal exploration because of *ascites* (accumulation of fluid in the peritoneum).

Symptoms and signs

The patient is usually comfortable, having no difficulty with breathing and complaining only of abdominal swelling, due to the ascites. Oedema may occur eventually. The liver will be enlarged and tender.

The jugular venous pressure is considerably raised, it may rise even higher in inspiration (*paradoxical venous pulsation*), and may show a steep 'y' descent (see p. 121) due to rapid early ventricular filling. The arterial pulse tends to be of small volume and is paradoxical. There may be tachycardia and, eventually, atrial fibrillation. An early third heart sound (*pericardial knock*) may be heard coinciding with the rapid filling of the right ventricle

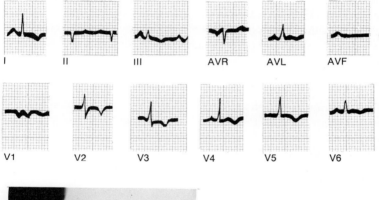

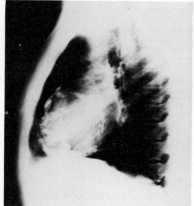

Figure 83 Chronic constrictive pericarditis

and the steep 'y' descent in the venous pulse. The electrocardiogram (Figure 83) shows the widespread inverted T waves of chronic pericarditis.

Chest X-rays show a normal or slightly large heart, sometimes with a shell of calcium in the pericardium around the heart. This is very suggestive of a tuberculous aetiology (cause). A small heart on X-ray, in what appears to be severe congestive heart failure, suggests the possibility of constrictive pericarditis. Cardiac catheterization is not usually necessary for diagnosis, but shows characteristic features.

Treatment
Mild cases are best left alone. More severe ones may be helped with digoxin and diuretics, but most will need surgical removal of the thick pericardium. Provided diagnosis is made early, operative mortality should not be more than 5 per cent. Of those who survive, the results are excellent. *Re-constriction* occurs in a few, but most remain well and, in many, the venous pressure falls to normal.

The myocardium

The myocardium is the heart muscle which contracts and acts as the pump. The tissue is made up of a collection of long cells running parallel to each other, forming fibres. These cells have many lateral projections which used to be thought to connect with other cells to form an *anatomical syncytium*, but electron-microscope studies have shown that this is not so.

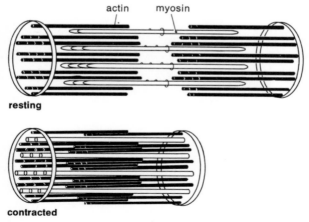

Figure 84 Interleafing of actin and myosin in a muscle fibre

The contraction of the muscle is brought about by the structure of the *sarcomere*. This is the functioning unit of the muscle cell, whose construction allows it to shorten itself. It is composed of two kinds of protein filament, *actin* and *myosin*, which are interleaved (Figure 84). The actin filaments are attached to membranes called *Z-lines*. As the actin filaments slide over the myosin filaments, the Z-lines are brought closer together, and this shortens the muscle cell. This process enables the heart to contract and drive its contents into the great blood vessels. As the sarcomere is progressively lengthened, so the force of contraction increases, and the heart can drive out more blood during systole. *Starling's law* (Figure 85) states that the greater the volume of the heart at the end of diastole, the greater will be the force of the following contraction.

The volume of the heart is related to the length of the sarcomere. As the sarcomere is stretched more, the force of contraction increases. However, there comes a point when it is stretched too much and the force decreases. The more force that is generated, the more blood the heart will be able to drive out during systole. The energy needed for the contraction is obtained by the oxidation of certain substances, such as glucose and fatty acids, to produce high-energy substances, such as creatine phosphate and adenosine triphosphate.

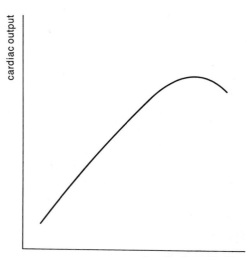

length of muscle fibre

Figure 85 Starling's law

The skeleton of the heart is formed by four rings of dense fibrous tissue which surround the four valves of the heart. To this skeleton are attached the atria at the top, the pulmonary artery, the aorta and the mitral and tricuspid valves. These two valves are also attached to the papillary muscles of the ventricles by the *chordae tendineae*. The ventricles, composed of sheets of muscle fibres arranged in a spiral manner, are attached to the lower surface of the fibrous skeleton. Thus, in each systole, the ventricles are literally 'wrung out', and little blood remains at the end.

Heart muscle disease

It was once thought that unexplained heart failure was due to either ischaemic heart disease (Chapter 3) that had not caused myocardial infarction or angina, or to hypertension (Chapter 5) after the blood pressure had fallen owing to heart failure or changes in heart muscle. These situations do occur, but there are other common causes. Some patients may have a primary disease of the myocardium itself. Many more have a myocardial disease which is secondary to a cause other than coronary artery disease or hypertension. Myocardial disease (*cardiomyopathy*) is divided into four main groups. However, it may be very difficult to determine exactly into which group a patient fits, and the patient may move from one group to another as the disease progresses. The four groups are as follows:

Congestive. The patient presents with a large heart in congestive cardiac failure. The pump fails to properly eject blood from the ventricles.

Restrictive. The heart is not so large, and the heart muscle cannot contract properly. The clinical picture is like that of constrictive pericarditis.

Hypertrophic. There is inappropriate hypertrophy of heart muscle, which cannot relax normally and interferes with ventricular filling in diastole.

Obliterative. A cardiac chamber is filled in by the disease process, as the right ventricle may be in endomyocardial fibrosis. In many cases, no specific cause may be found and indeed a simple classification is into primary, where no cause is known, and secondary, where the cause is known.

Some of these will now be described.

Myocarditis

This is inflammation of heart muscle. Known causes are rheumatic fever and diphtheria. Many infections may cause mild myocarditis, which goes unnoticed, but the disease may be more severe and lead to permanent damage in some viral infections, such as Coxsackie B virus, poliomyelitis and influenza. It may also occur in parasitic infestation such as Chagas' disease (South American trypanosomiasis) and toxoplasmosis. Some patients may show only electrocardiographic changes, while others suffer tachycardia, abnormal heart rhythms, and frank congestive failure. They may recover completely or be left with permanent damage causing a form of congestive cardiomyopathy.

Infiltrative cardiomyopathy

In some diseases the myocardium may be infiltrated, giving rise to a 'restrictive' or to a 'congestive' picture. Examples are amyloidosis, scleroderma and haemochromatosis.

Tropical cardiomyopathy

Particular types of heart muscle disease have been described in South Africa and Jamaica, but the best known is *endomyocardial fibrosis*, which is very common in East and West Africa. The cause is unknown. Fibrous tissue is deposited in the apex of the right ventricle and on the left ventricular wall. It presents a clinical picture much like that of constrictive pericarditis on the right and, on the left, of mitral regurgitation going on to secondary pulmonary arterial hypertension and heart failure. It may be very difficult to distinguish from tuberculous constrictive pericarditis or from rheumatic mitral regurgitation.

Toxic cardiomyopathy

Alcohol is thought to cause heart muscle disease, and some drugs such as *emetine* and *antimony* are also known to damage the myocardium, although this is usually temporary. An epidemic of cardiomyopathy in Canada was found to have been caused by cobalt in beer.

Secondary cardiomyopathy

Heart muscle disease may occasionally occur during, or following, pregnancy. It has also been found in cases of cirrhosis of the liver and in some diseases of the nervous system, such as Friedreich's ataxia and the muscular dystrophies. Any heart muscle disease occurring in a known generalized disease is considered 'secondary'.

Familial cardiomyopathy

Heart enlargement that runs in families has been known for many years. A recently found disease which is a good example of obstructive cardiomyopathy is *hypertrophic obstructive cardiomyopathy*, also known as *idiopathic hypertrophic sub-aortic stenosis*. In this condition, the heart muscle hypertrophies, particularly the interventricular septum. This may obstruct the flow of blood into and out of the ventricles. However, the essential features are hypertrophy of the heart muscle fibres and a resistance to diastolic filling. The cause of this disease is unknown, although there is a family history of it in about half the cases. It is usually most marked on the left side. It may occur at any age and in both sexes.

Patients may suffer angina because of the inability of the coronary circulation to adequately oxygenate the excessive mass of muscle, they may experience breathlessness, loss of consciousness on exertion, and a peculiar liability to sudden death. The pulse is jerky because of the rapid ejection of blood by the thick ventricle, followed by sudden diminution of flow as the walls of the ventricles come together and obstruct the flow. The left ventricle is felt to be powerful, an atrial sound can be heard and an atrial beat felt. There is a late systolic murmur as the obstruction occurs. The electrocardiogram shows a good deal of left ventricular hypertrophy. However, the patient may present with no murmurs and no evidence of obstruction even with a 'congestive' picture.

The outlook is poor, and treatment is difficult. Propranolol may reduce cardiac work and relieve the angina, but it probably does not improve the prognosis. Surgical treatment, resecting wedges of muscle (mostly from the septum) to relieve the obstruction, is sometimes attempted.

Heart transplantation

In the future, some of the severe forms of ischaemic heart disease and cardiomyopathies, in intractible heart failure where there is virtually no heart muscle left, may be treated by heart transplant (Figure 86) or the insertion of an artificial heart. The success of kidney transplants raised hopes that heart transplants would also be possible. Unfortunately, the rejection of foreign tissue has been more severe with the heart than with the kidney. In the heart, the rejection has been associated with the obliteration of the blood vessels in the transplant, denying it nourishment and leading to ischaemia, fibrosis and calcification. Eventually, the transplant

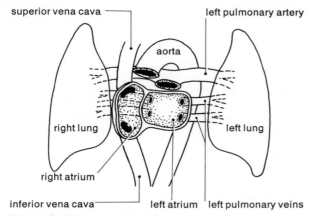

Figure 86 Heart transplantation.
The diagram shows the remnant of the recipient heart to which the donor heart is joined at transplanting

becomes useless and the patient dies. In spite of the use of drugs such as azathioprine, steroids and antilymphocytic serum to suppress the immune reaction that rejects the transplant, in spite of careful tissue typing and donor selection, and in spite of nursing the patient in a sterile, air-conditioned cubicle, this problem has not been overcome. The surgical progress has been considerable, and many of the technical difficulties have been overcome. Of the first 120 heart transplants, 17 per cent lived for six months or longer.

Much work continues, but it is not possible to say whether the answer will be artificial hearts or transplanted human hearts. If these operations become feasible, the more severe and complex kinds of congenital heart diseases might also be helped. If heart and lung transplants become possible, then congenital hearts with the Eisenmenger syndrome and diseased lung blood vessels (see p. 132) could also be helped.

The endocardium

The endocardium is the inner layer of the heart consisting of a single layer of simple squamous epithelium supported by a layer of fibro–elastic connective tissue. The heart valves are also formed of endocardium and are covered on both surfaces with endothelium. The main endocardial disease is infection of the endocardium of the heart valves, although the endocardium is also involved in other diseases: commonly in rheumatic heart diseases, endomyocardial fibrosis common in tropical Africa and fibro-elastosis, which is seen in some congenital heart disease in infants.

Acute infective endocarditis

This is usually part of an overwhelming septicaemia, and the infection of heart valves may not be recognized before the post-mortem room. Previously normal heart valves may be invaded and destroyed, so that murmurs will appear that were not previously present. If the situation is diagnosed sufficiently early, a response to suitable antibiotics is possible. However, many patients die of overwhelming infection and heart failure. Organisms such as *Staphylococcus aureus*, *Neisseria gonorrhoeae* and *Streptococcus pyogenes* have been incriminated. Despite the division into acute and subacute, there is a considerable range of severity, from overwhelming and acute to subacute and chronic. All are potentially lethal, and demand treatment as rapidly as a diagnosis can be made. Even in the least virulent infections, delay may be fatal.

Subacute infective endocarditis

This is also known as *subacute bacterial endocarditis* and is applied to the more common variety of endocarditis when the organism infecting the heart is less virulent, and the progress of the disease insidious. The heart is usually abnormal, but the abnormality is often so minor that the patient, and indeed the doctor, may be quite unaware of it. The heart abnormalities which tend to become infected are mild mitral regurgitation, aortic regurgitation, small ventricular septal defects, persistent ductus arteriosus, congenital bicuspid aortic valve, pulmonary stenosis, coarctation of the aorta and any kind of surgically replaced valve. In congenital abnormalities with little turbulence of blood flow, such as in atrial septal defect, infection is uncommon.

Usually any organisms that get into the blood stream are rapidly killed by the body's defence mechanism but, if the endocardium is damaged, they may find a niche in it where they can survive and multiply. Platelets, fibrin, organisms, blood cells and dead tissue form vegetations which look like clusters of small grapes. These are likely to break off, and are responsible for many features of the disease. The most common organism is *Streptococcus viridans*, followed by *Streptococcus faecalis*. However, many other bacteria may infect the heart in this way and occasionally *Rickettsiae* (*R. Burneti*) and fungi may also do so.

Symptoms

These often occur so gradually and are so vague that their importance
may be missed, particularly in old people. Short courses of antibiotics may
temporarily suppress the infection and make diagnosis more difficult.

In over half the patients a possible source of infection may be identified.
Many of those with *Streptococcus viridans* infections have had teeth
extracted or scaled before the symptoms started. Organisms easily get in
to the blood system after such treatment, but they are quickly destroyed,
even in patients with heart disease. However, if the endocardium is
damaged, the organisms may survive there and give rise to the disease.
There may be a history of preceding surgery, usually on the gut, in the
pelvis or on the urinary tract. Even cystoscopy may cause an infection
from *Streptococcus faecalis* or *Enterococcus*. The patient may have an
artificial heart valve. This disease can sometimes be found in the
previously normal heart. For example, a drug addict repeatedly injecting
himself using dirty needles and syringes may get septicaemia and may
develop staphylococcal endocarditis of the (presumably normal) tricuspid
valve, resulting then in severe tricuspid regurgitation.

The patient may feel general malaise, vague ill health, loss of weight and
appetite, unusual sweating, vague aches and pains, and may think it is
influenza. The patient may present with a complication due to an
embolus caused by one of the vegetations breaking off. The symptoms
may be abdominal pain from an embolus to the spleen, kidney or gut,
hemiplegia (paralysis of one side of the body) from a cerebral embolus,
loss of vision from a retinal embolus or chest pain from a pulmonary or
coronary embolus. The patient may be breathless, and this will worsen if
heart failure occurs or the strain on the heart increases due to the gradual
destruction of the valve.

On clinical examination, a number of features may be found, although
they seldom occur all together. The patient may be mildly anaemic
owing to the infection and often has a low-grade fever. Any patient who
is vaguely ill and whose anaemia cannot be explained may be suffering
from this disease. Crops of small red streaks (*splinter haemorrhages*) may be
found under the nails and small tender raised swellings (*Osler's nodes*) in
the pulps of the fingers and toes due to emboli in the small vessels. Small
haemorrhages caused by emboli may be seen in the conjunctivae and with
an ophthalmoscope in the retina. Sometimes, large tender swellings
occur in the limbs. Pulsation in an artery such as the radial artery may
disappear if it is obstructed by an embolus, and may give rise to an

aneurysm (bulge) of the vessel. Moderate clubbing of the fingers is a valuable sign, and appears within a few weeks of the infection. The spleen is often enlarged and can be felt. Because of emboli to the kidney, red blood cells are commonly seen on microscopic examination of the urine. Signs of heart disease are usually found, though less often in elderly people. There may only be a soft systolic murmur, which gets louder or changes as the valve tissue is destroyed and the heart lesion worsens.

Diagnosis
This depends on blood culture, although it is helped if a modestly raised white blood count from an increase in the neutrophils (the most common type of white cell), a raised E S R, anaemia, or red cells in the urine are found. Blood should be taken for culture several times a day for a few successive days, particularly at the time of fever. It is inoculated on plates of several different media in order to identify the infecting organism. However, even before the organism has grown, it will be necessary to start the treatment. In 60–90 per cent of cases, it will be possible to grow an organism on one of the plates, and the sensitivity of this organism to different antibiotics can then be assessed in order to guide treatment.

However, in some cases it may not be possible to identify the organism, and the clinical diagnosis will be the only guide to treatment. If there is a reasonable suspicion that the patient is suffering from this disease, he must be given a full course of treatment since, if it is present and is not treated, he will almost certainly die.

Treatment
The most important antibiotic for the treatment of this disease is *penicillin* (Figure 87), unless the blood-culture tests suggest it is unsuitable. A large dose (10–20 million units daily) is needed and it is given as the potassium salt, since too much sodium may precipitate heart failure. A venous catheter is used and the penicillin is put into 1 litre of 5 per cent glucose containing 50 mg heparin to prevent clotting, and 5 mg hydrocortisone to suppress inflammation around the tube. If the patient is in bed, an automatic drip regulator can be used. When necessary, the catheter is changed to a new vein. If the patient is well enough, he can wheel his drip stand about with him, but he may need reassurance that the drip tube will not come out.

Streptomycin (1 g per day) is sometimes added to the infusion, but it may have serious and permanent toxic effects such as vertigo and deafness, so the blood level should be watched. In a few cases probenecid (2 g per day) is used to keep a high level of penicillin in the blood stream by blocking its excretion by the kidneys.

The treatment is continued for six weeks initially. When the organism is grown, sensitivity tests may occasionally indicate that it is completely insensitive to penicillin. Then other antibiotics, such as methicillin, cloxacillin, ampicillin, cephaloridine and fucidin may be used. Drugs which only suppress the bacteria (*bacteriostatic*), such as tetracycline and chloramphenicol, are seldom used as they do not lead to complete control. Penicillin and other bactericidal drugs actually kill the invading organisms. Close cooperation between the clinician and the microbiologist is essential in choosing the correct drugs.

Fungal infections are very difficult to treat. Amphotericin B may be used. Endocarditis may occur after Q fever, from infection with

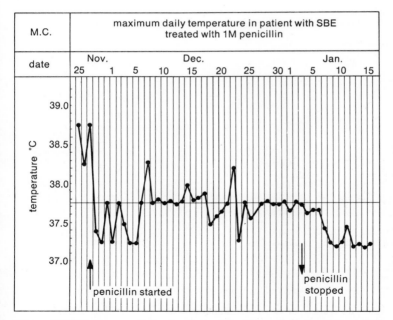

Figure 87 Temperature chart of patient with subacute infective endocarditis, showing response to penicillin treatment

R. Burneti. This might be suspected if no organism was identified in the blood cultures, the aortic valve was affected and there was no response to treatment. It may be possible to find antibodies in the blood, which helps in diagnosis. Treatment is a very long course of tetracycline, although this is often ineffective. If the infection cannot be controlled, or so much damage has been done that there is danger of heart failure, it may be necessary to replace the aortic valve. Even in bacteriological infections, if the disease cannot be controlled with antibiotics, then surgical replacement of the infected valve may be necessary. A valve may also have to be replaced because it has been destroyed and is inefficient. If a transplanted valve becomes infected, it is often necessary to remove it and put in another.

After an adequate course of treatment, when the patient feels better, the fever has gone and the ESR is normal, repeat blood cultures are carried out. Several will be necessary but, if all are negative, the patient is probably cured. Even so, the patient should be watched for any sign of recurrence, when more blood cultures would be taken and the treatment repeated.

Hospital No..

....has a

Heart disorder, and is under the care of

Prof./Dr. ....

ANTIBIOTIC COVER is required
under the following circumstances
A. TO PREVENT BACTERIAL ENDOCARDITIS:

I. DENTAL EXTRACTIONS OR SCALING
(Penicillin * I mega μ I.M.)
30 minutes before operation, followed by
Phenoxymethyl penicillin (penicillin V) 250 mgm.
4 times daily (or equivalent) for three days by
mouth, or for as long as any infection persists.

* For patients allergic to penicillin
Cephaloridine 500 mg. should be given instead
(250 mg. for children)

YOU SHOULD VISIT YOUR DENTIST REGULARLY

2. OTHER SEPSIS
Tonsilitis (oral Penicillin for one week)

Respiratory Infections
(Tetracycline, or ampicillin for one week)

3. SURGICAL PROCEDURES
Any potentially septic operation particularly
instrumentation of the bladder or rectum
(Penicillin and Streptomycin)

4. CHILDBIRTH
(Penicillin and Streptomycin)

B. TO PREVENT A RECURRENCE OF
RHEUMATIC FEVER

Sulphadimidine 0.5Gm. twice daily should be
taken by mouth indefinitely

Figure 88 Card to be carried by all patients with organic heart disease

In most patients the infection can be controlled, but the death rate is unfortunately about 30 per cent. These deaths are due to the effects of the infection on the heart, the embolic complications, worsening of the heart lesion and heart failure. The earlier the diagnosis can be made, the greater the chance of success.

Prevention

Any patient with a heart lesion, however trivial, must obtain adequate antibiotic cover for all dental treatment, for all operations however minor and to cover childbirth. He should also carry a card (Figure 88). Susceptible heart abnormalities should be corrected as early as possible. Ventricular septal defects should be closed, a persistent ductus arteriosus ligated and coarctation of the aorta resected. These operations may be needed even when infections are present, in order to bring them under control.

Summary of nursing points

The heart is perhaps the most vital part of the body. It consists of the pericardium, the myocardium and the endocardium – all these structures are subject to disease.

The nurse should understand common pathological conditions that affect the heart – pericarditis, myocarditis and endocarditis – together with their clinical manifestations, investigations, prevention and treatment.

The nursing care of the patient with heart disease is vital in ensuring his recovery. Important points are nursing position and ensuring that the correct diet and medication is given as prescribed. The patient is usually nursed in bed in the most comfortable position. Lifting and moving of the patient should always be done by two nurses. The patient should have his pressure areas treated regularly and oxygen should be given as prescribed.

Nursing observations must include temperature, pulse, respiration, blood pressure, fluid balance, bowels, skin and the emotional state of the patient. Accurate records must be kept of these observations and any change in the patient's condition should be noted and promptly recorded and remedial action taken.

Chapter 10

Diseases of the arteries and veins

The anatomy of the systemic arteries

The main channel of blood supply for the whole body is the *aorta* (Figures 89 and 90). This arises from the left ventricle of the heart and as it leaves the heart it is known as the *ascending aorta*. It gives off the *right* and *left coronary arteries* almost immediately. It curves over to the left, becoming the *arch of the aorta* and gives off the *innominate artery*, which soon divides into the *right subclavian artery* that supplies the right upper limb and the *right common carotid artery* that supplies the head and neck.

The aorta then gives off the *left common carotid artery*, which also supplies the head and the neck, and then the *left subclavian artery*, which supplies the left upper limb. It then arches down into the thorax as the *descending aorta*, and gives rise to the *bronchial arteries*, which supply the tissue of the lung with arterial blood and allow the lungs their double blood supply; it also gives rise to the *intercostal arteries*. The descending aorta passes into the abdomen through a hole in the diaphragm to become the *abdominal aorta*. Here it gives rise to the great *coeliac artery* which divides into its *left gastric*, *splenic* and *hepatic* branches supplying the stomach, spleen and liver.

The next major artery is the *superior mesenteric artery*, which supplies the gut and then the two *renal arteries* left and right to the kidneys. The *inferior mesenteric artery* supplies the lower gut. The abdominal aorta terminates by dividing into the right and left *common iliac* arteries which in turn divide into the *internal and external iliac arteries*. The internal iliac arteries supply the pelvic organs, and the external iliac artery passes under the inguinal ligament to become the *femoral artery*. This soon gives off the *profunda femoris artery* to the thigh muscles. In the popliteal fossa below the knee joint, it becomes the *popliteal artery* which divides into the *posterior and anterior tibial arteries* to the legs and finally to the feet, the anterior tibial artery becoming the *dorsalis pedis* on the dorsum of the foot (Figure 90).

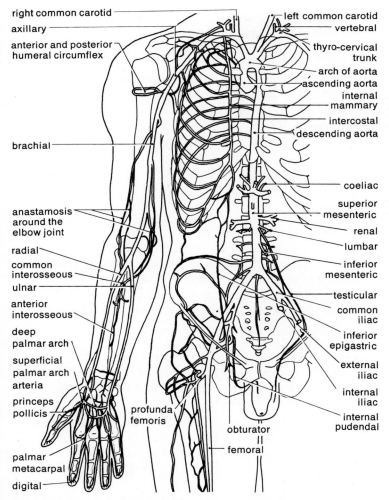

right common carotid
axillary
anterior and posterior
humeral circumflex

brachial

anastamosis
around the
elbow joint

radial
common
interosseous
ulnar

anterior
interosseous

deep
palmar arch

superficial
palmar arch
arteria

princeps
pollicis

palmar
metacarpal

digital

profunda
femoris

obturator

femoral

left common carotid
vertebral

thyro-cervical
trunk
arch of aorta
ascending aorta
internal
mammary
intercostal
descending aorta

coeliac

superior
mesenteric

renal
lumbar

inferior
mesenteric

testicular
common
iliac

inferior
epigastric

external
iliac

internal
iliac

internal
pudendal

Figure 89 Distribution of the major systemic arteries

The *subclavian arteries* become the *axillary arteries* and then the *brachial arteries* to the arms. These in turn divide at the elbow into the *radial* and *ulnar arteries* to the forearm and finally to the hand.

The walls of the larger arteries are made up of elastic tissue and muscle, controlled by the sympathetic nervous system. They can stretch and can vary their width to control the peripheral vascular resistance and the flow of blood. Thus, when a vital organ such as the brain needs more blood, this can be ensured, although it is at the expense of tissues such as the skin which can, however, manage with very little blood.

The anatomy of the veins

The veins drain the blood from the areas supplied by the arteries, and return it to the heart. On the whole, they accompany the arteries (Figures 90 and 91), but there are different arrangements in the head and in the portal system. The walls of veins are thin, and have no muscle or elastic fibres. However, unlike arteries, veins contain valves so that, once blood has moved forward, it cannot go back. The forward movement of blood is largely brought about by the constant contraction and relaxation of the muscles (the '*muscle pump*').

Disease of the aorta

The aorta is a large blood vessel, about 3 cm in diameter. It has three coats: the inner one, the *intima*, is a simple lining of endothelial cells; the middle one, the *media*, is composed of muscle and elastic tissue which enable it to even out blood flow and pressures; and the outer one, the *adventitia*, is composed of fibrous tissue and serves to strengthen the aorta so it can withstand the high pressures to which it is subjected.

There are several causes of disease of the aorta:

1 *Atherosclerosis*. This is a degenerative process which involves most arteries to differing degrees as people get older. It is described in relation to the coronary arteries on page 39. In the aorta, it tends to weaken the wall rather than obstruct the lumen.

2 *Syphilis*. This is a very common cause of aortic disease in some parts of the world, although now much less so in the West. It occurs in the later stages of syphilis, and mostly affects the ascending aorta. Inflammation and narrowing of the small blood vessels that nourish the aortic wall result in an inadequate blood supply to its deeper tissues, and these die and are replaced by fibrous tissue. Once fibrosed, it is stronger

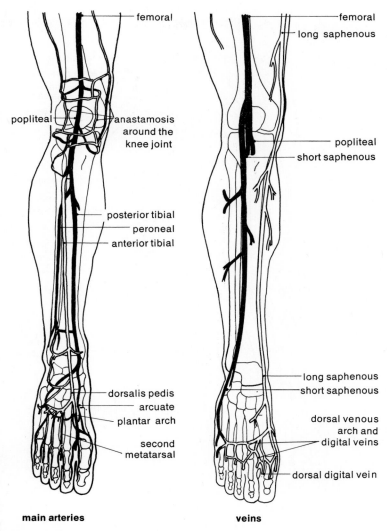

main arteries

veins

Figure 90 Major blood vessels of the leg and foot

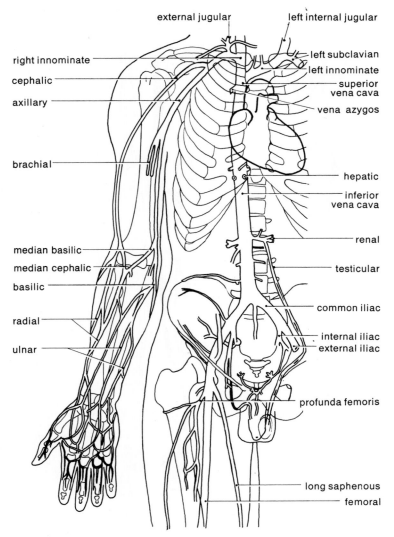

Figure 91 Distribution of the major veins

than a normal aorta, but before this occurs it is weaker and may stretch. The diseased tissue eventually calcifies, and the thin parallel lines of calcium in the ascending aorta seen on a chest X-ray are diagnostic of syphilitic aortic disease.

3 *Trauma*. Rupture of the aorta from the sudden deceleration of a car crash is not uncommon. The vessel is fixed at certain points and tends to tear near them. In most instances the aorta ruptures into the pericardium and there is almost immediate death from cardiac tamponade (see p. 160). However, in a few cases fibrous tissue is able to contain the blood for a while and in these patients surgical treatment may be successful.

4 *Congenital*. In an abnormality of the muscular coat of the aorta known as *cystic medial necrosis*, the elastic fibres degenerate and are replaced with starchy material. This is probably a congenital biochemical fault, and the condition may be associated with other congenital abnormalities, such as coarctation of the aorta or with *Marfan's syndrome* of abnormally long fingers (*arachnodactyly*) and long limbs, dislocated lenses of the eyes, an abnormally high hard palate and poor muscular tone. The changes in the aorta may only be discovered as an incidental finding at post mortem, or they may lead to dissecting aneurysm (see below), often precipitated by pregnancy or hypertension.

5 *Mycotic*. This is caused by an infected embolus which, in infective endocarditis, may break away from the affected part of the heart and lodge on the wall of the aorta.

6 *Other causes*. Reiter's disease (urethritis, conjunctivitis and arthritis) and ankylosing spondylitis, both of unknown cause, may be associated with disease of the aorta and its complications.

Since the aorta is subjected to the considerable pressure of blood ejected from the powerful left ventricle, it tends to rupture or stretch if it is diseased. Rupture is usually fatal. Stretch leads to what is called an *aneurysm*, of which there are several different kinds.

Dissecting aneurysm

This is associated with a defective medial coat of the aorta, and usually cystic medial necrosis. It is more likely to occur if the patient is hypertensive, and may also be seen in pregnancy. The aorta tears on the inside, usually just above the aortic valve, and blood tracks between the coats of the aorta. This may spread along branches of the aorta, including

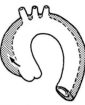

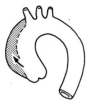

Type I   **Type II**

Figure 92 Dissecting aneurysms

those of the arch and even down to the renal and iliac arteries. It may block the coronary arteries, and also involve the aortic valve to cause aortic regurgitation. The aorta may rupture externally which will usually kill the patient, or it may rupture back into the aorta, the patient occasionally surviving. Where the dissecting aneurysm is confined to the ascending aorta, it is known as Type II, if it extends beyond this, it is Type I (Figure 92).

Symptoms and signs
Usually very severe 'tearing' pain is felt in the chest, front and back, and sometimes in the abdomen. It may settle down, only to recur later, and may be felt in other places if the dissection continues into other branches of the aorta and blocks them. The patient is pale and sweating with a rapid pulse rate. Some normally palpable arterial pulses may be missing. An aortic diastolic murmur may occasionally be heard. The electrocardiogram does not help, but a chest X-ray may show widening of the upper mediastinal shadow. X-rays taken after the injection of radio-opaque due into the aorta may confirm the diagnosis and show the extent of the dissection. It may be difficult to distinguish this disease from myocardial infarction.

The outlook is very poor. About 20 per cent of patients die within a few hours and almost all others within a week. About 15 per cent recover spontaneously, although they still have a permanently dissected aorta.

Treatment
In the acute stage, the treatment is medical. The blood pressure should be quickly lowered to about 100 mmHg systolic using hypotensive drugs systemically, and then these drugs can be given by mouth. Diamorphine may well be needed to control the pain. If the patient survives, surgical treatment may be undertaken to resect the diseased aorta and replace it

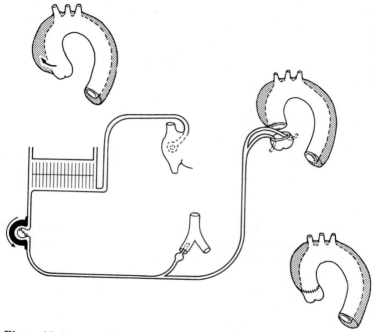

Figure 93 Surgery of Type I dissecting aneurysm.
The aorta is divided at the level of the intimal tear, oversewing the double lumen
distally and re-anastamosing the aorta; blood is thus directed into the true lumen

with a Dacron graft; with a Type II dissecting aneurysm, the ascending
aorta is replaced in this way. Other operations are sometimes carried
out, such as to oversew the double lumen and thus direct the blood back
into its proper channel; this is particularly used for a Type I dissecting
aneurysm (Figure 93).

Saccular and fusiform aneurysms

These are more localized than dissecting aneurysms. They are called
fusiform if the entire circumference of the aorta is involved, and *saccular*
if only part is involved.

Any of the diseases of the aortic wall already described may cause these
aneurysms. There are often no symptoms, and they may be a chance
finding on a routine chest X-ray. However, the aneurysms may press on
surrounding structures such as the bronchi (where they cause wheezing)
the oesophagus (where they cause difficulty in swallowing) the bones (pain)

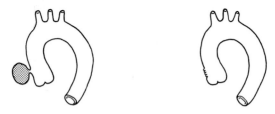

Figure 94 Saccular aneurysm – excision and repair

or the recurrent laryngeal nerve (hoarseness). There are usually no physical signs, but occasionally an aneurysm may be large enough to cause pulsation of the chest wall, or 'tug' the trachea with each heart beat as it pushes down the left main bronchus.

Although the patient may live for many years, most die within two. Death is from rupture of the aneurysm or from an associated cause such as hypertension, ischaemic heart disease or a stroke. Surgical treatment is considered if the aneurysm is larger or is getting larger or is causing symptoms. Saccular aneurysms are excised and the aorta repaired (Figure 94). Age, in itself, is no bar to surgery, particularly if the patient has the common atherosclerotic aneurysms of the abdominal aorta. However, if the coronary and cerebral circulations are not functioning adequately, such treatment should not be considered. With a fusiform aneurysm, it is usually necessary to resect the diseased aorta and to replace it with a Dacron graft (Figure 95). Grafts of human aorta, obtained at autopsy and specially prepared, can also be used.

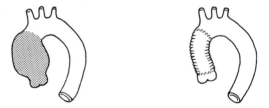

Figure 95 Fusiform aneurysm of the ascending aorta – excision and grafting

Peripheral arterial disease

This is mostly due to degenerative atheromatous change. The effects of this on the coronary arteries are described on page 39. In this chapter, we shall concentrate on atherosclerosis in the iliac vessels and the lower limbs.

Intermittent claudication

This means intermittent limping, and was originally observed in horses. It is like angina of the legs and is a very common disease, particularly in elderly or middle-aged men. The most common complaint is of pain, in one or both calves, when walking. Usually it brings the patient to a stop and rapidly improves on standing still, only to recur on walking again. It is usually described as a cramp. The distance that can be walked varies and indicates the degree of obstruction to blood flow in the legs. The leg muscles are not getting sufficient oxygen. Occasionally the pain involves only the muscles of the feet; or it may be more extensive and involve the muscles of the thigh and buttocks, which implies that there is a block at the level of the common iliac arteries. Much more rarely, it may occur in the upper limb and the patient may be unable to write.

Eventually there may be pain even when the patient is resting, and this is a very serious situation. The patient may have to sit on the bed with his legs hanging down to get any relief at all. Hypertension, ischaemic heart disease and diabetes mellitus are quite often associated with atheromatous disease of the lower limbs.

The skin colour of an ischaemic limb may appear unduly pale, and colour returns abnormally slowly after the blanching caused by pressing it with a finger. If the leg is lifted up, the arterial pressure is inadequate to drive blood through the narrowed arteries, and the leg rapidly becomes deathly white. If it is then allowed to hang over the edge of the bed, the colour returns only slowly and in a patchy fashion, the leg eventually becoming a rather cyanotic red. Because of the poor blood supply, the pulps of the toes tend to waste away and the hairs disappear. Eventually, the skin may become abnormally thin and shiny, may lacerate and become gangrenous. The peripheral pulses may be weak or non-existent. If the disease is at all severe, the dorsalis pedis and posterior popliteal pulses are usually absent. The femoral pulses may be weak or absent if the block is in the iliac arteries or higher. A systolic murmur may be heard over a partially blocked vessel.

Treatment

Drugs are commonly used in the hope that they will dilate the affected vessels, but they are usually ineffective because of the permanent damage already done to the vessel walls. Some patients can benefit enormously from a programme of graduated exercise. They walk a slightly longer distance each day, either by normal walking or on a treadmill, gradually improving their 'claudication distance'. The programme needs careful control, with constant encouragement to the patient.

Surgery is considered for any severe case, particularly for the younger patients, but careful investigation is needed first. Arteriography can be carried out by passing a catheter through the femoral artery into the popliteal artery and injecting radio-opaque dye. X-rays will then show the anatomy of the arterial tree, exposing any irregularity of the vessels and any blockage. This will show whether operation is possible, and help plan the procedure. The diseased inner tissue can be stripped out with instruments or carbon dioxide under pressure. A graft can be inserted using an artery, a vein or a plastic substitute like Dacron. Sometimes it may be necessary to graft at a high level to replace the lower abdominal aorta and the common iliac arteries. These operations are very successful.

The care of the chronic ischaemic limb
If operation is impossible and general care is exercised, the limb may remain reasonably healthy for a long while. Cleanliness is most important. The feet should be washed in warm water every day. They should be carefully dried and then spirit applied to them. After this has evaporated, they should be powered with a good talc. Any infection such as athlete's foot should be treated. The feet should be kept at a constant and reasonable temperature, avoiding extremes of heat or cold. Treatment by a chiropodist is often better than clumsy efforts to cut nails and pare corns. Shoes should be comfortable and should not rub or exert undue pressure anywhere. Any suggestion of a scratch should be treated seriously. Bacterial infections will need an antibiotic, taken by mouth. At night, the legs should be slightly lower than the rest of the body. If a patch of gangrene develops, this should usually be carefully removed by a surgeon. Smoking undoubtedly worsens this condition and should be discouraged unless the patient is very elderly.

Peripheral arterial embolism

This is likely to cause more trouble in the lower than the upper limb. The embolus may be a piece of atherosclerotic tissue that has broken off, but is usually thrombus from the heart. It may come from the left atrium in mitral stenosis with atrial fibrillation (see p. 99), or from the left ventricle after myocardial infarction (see p. 49) or in cardiomyopathy (see p. 166). It may come from a valve with infective endocarditis (see p. 171) or from a tumour in the left atrium.

The symptoms are sudden. The leg becomes painful, cold and white, and the pulses are absent. There may be spontaneous recovery which will, however, often leave disabling intermittent claudication; but usually surgical removal of the embolus is needed. This is an emergency, but there is time to prepare the patient and get him into a fit condition. Anticoagulants are usually used such as heparin or *thrombokinase* intravenously, then warfarin by mouth. Ideally, the embolus is removed with Fogarty's catheter. This is a catheter with a small balloon at its tip, which is passed along the artery. The balloon is then blown up and drawn back, bringing with it any debris and the clot in the artery. This is a highly successful procedure.

Thromboangiitis obliterans (Buerger's disease)

This curious disease affects the arteries and veins of men between the ages of twenty-five and forty. These patients usually smoke excessively. The vessels are involved in a non-atheromatous obliterative process, associated with thrombus formation. Histologically, it is an inflammation. It tends to occur in attacks, and there may be years between them. Superficial thrombophlebitis is common. Involvement of the arteries of the lower limbs causes intermittent claudication. Later, the upper limbs may also be involved, and *Raynaud's phenomenon* may occur. Treatment is not very satisfactory and follows that described above (see p. 185). It is often necessary to amputate the limb. The patients should be stopped from smoking.

Raynaud's phenomenon

This is caused by a spasm of the small arterioles in the fingers, and occurs less commonly in the toes, nose and ears. It is mostly related to cold, and some of the fingers become cyanotic or white (or both) and may be very painful. Mild attacks are easily relieved by warmth and massage, but severe ones may respond to nothing, the fingers becoming numb and clumsy. Pins and needles may occur during recovery.

If the attacks continue for years, permanent changes occur in the skin; it becomes shiny, the fingers become tapered from loss of tissue, and infections such as whitlows (*paronychia*) are common. Painful gangrenous ulcers may also occur. Eventually the bone may become involved, and the end of the finger may even break off.

A few cases have no apparent cause, and are called *Raynaud's disease*; the rest are secondary to some other disease, and are known as Raynaud's phenomenon. There are many causes: the most common is *scleroderma*, but the phenomenon also occurs in other collagen diseases such as systemic lupus erythematosus, rheumatoid arthritis and polyarteritis nodosa. Vibration may cause it, as happens with pneumatic-drill operators. It is sometimes caused by a cervical rib pressing on the nerves leaving the spinal foramina or by certain diseases of the nervous system, such as syringomyelia. It can result from syphilis or from a toxic substance, such as ergot, and is also seen in some blood disorders such as polycythaemia and haemolytic anaemia, and in generalized arterial disorders such as atherosclerosis and Buerger's disease.

Treatment is very unsatisfactory since, so far, no drug has been shown to bring relief. There are obvious general measures, such as wearing gloves to keep the hands warm. Sometimes a cause such as systemic lupus can be treated. *Sympathectomy* (the removal of the sympathetic fibres to the upper limb) can be carried out. All the blood vessels dilate and there is improvement but, unfortunately, it often only lasts a few months.

Deep venous thrombosis

This may occur at any time but is particularly liable to occur after any prolonged illness involving a stay in bed, surgical operation or childbirth. Venous thrombosis may be associated with a carcinoma, particularly of the bronchus or pancreas, or with the contraceptive pill, and it may occur without any apparent cause even in the young.

The danger with this disease is that thrombus may break off, become an embolus and be swept to the pulmonary artery, often killing the patient (see p. 148). A less dangerous, but very disabling, effect is that *varicose veins* may follow or that the valves in the veins may be destroyed, leading to persistent oedema.

If the thrombus is silent, produces neither symptoms nor signs and is only recognized when a complication occurs, it may be called *phlebothrombosis* but, if it presents with pain and swelling, it is called *thrombophlebitis*. There may be a little fever but the chief complaint is of a swollen, painful, often discoloured, limb. However, there may be only calf tenderness or perhaps just a positive *Homan's sign* (pain in the calf on forceful dorsiflexion of the foot). If not clinically obvious, the presence of deep venous thrombosis can be shown by a simple ultrasonic technique, and its extent demonstrated by injecting radio-opaque dye into the veins and taking X-ray pictures.

This is a common disease. Treatment is aimed at rapid resolution and the prevention of further thrombosis with its risk of embolism. Analgesics such as *paracetamol* may be needed in the early stages, but the basic treatment is continuous intravenous heparin controlled by clotting times, usually about 30 000 to 40 000 units in each 24 hours. There is often rapid improvement in pain and swelling, but the heparin should be continued for at least a week and then warfarin given for about three months. As soon as the patient feels better, he may begin to walk again, although he may need elastic stockings to control any residual oedema. If there are recurrent pulmonary emboli, it may sometimes be necessary to tie off or *plicate* (take a tuck in) the inferior vena cava, although the collateral vessels that form are just as dangerous, in the long term, in allowing emboli to pass. Prevention of this disease and the important role of the nurse are discussed on page 151.

Superficial venous thrombosis

A painful hard cord along the line of a superficial vein may occur without evidence of deep thrombosis (which may, nevertheless, be present). Superficial thrombophlebitis is treated in the same way as deep venous thrombosis and is potentially just as dangerous. Recurrent ('migratory') superficial phlebitis in different veins is often associated with malignant disease.

Varicose veins

These may be merely unsightly or there may be symptoms, such as aching legs. They may be associated with the oedema of venous insufficiency, with *eczema* or with frank *ulceration*. If they are not severe, the patient may be made more comfortable with simple measures such as elastic stockings. Other patients may need treatment with injections or compression techniques, or the veins may need to be stripped.

Summary of nursing points

The patency of the veins and arteries is vital in maintaining an effective circulation, thus ensuring the correct functioning of the body as a whole. Any disease, deformity or obstruction of these vessels may lead to a fatal result.

The nurse should understand the main pathological conditions, such as atherosclerosis, embolism, aneurysm, thrombosis and Raynaud's disease, together with their clinical manifestations, investigations and treatment.

She must also maintain accurate observations and records. She must ensure scrupulous cleanliness of ischaemic limbs, because of the possibility of tissue breakdown and infection. As the danger of gangrene is great, special precautions must be taken to prevent damage to the skin. For example, careful toilet of the feet should be carried out, extremes of temperature of the water used for bathing should be avoided and the skin must be thoroughly dried on completion.

Further reading

General
Books

S. Alstead, A. G. Macgregor and R. H. Girdwood (eds.), *Textbook of Medical Treatment*, 12th edn, Churchill Livingstone, 1971. Chapters 4 and 5 are relevant and provide a clear, comprehensive description of cardiovascular disorders, their features and management.

P. M. Ashworth and H. Rose, *Cardiovascular Disorders: Patient Care*. Baillière Tindall, 1973. A comprehensive account of the nursing of patients with these disorders and the facts necessary to understand and enjoy that nursing.

R. Barrymore, *Practical Diet for Heart Disease*, Arthur Barker, 1964. A very simple guide to healthy eating, with special reference to the effect of food on heart disease.

P. F. Binnion, *A Short Textbook of Chemical Physiology*, Lloyd-Luke, 1969. Chapter 3 applies physiology to the disorders of the cardiovascular system and to the investigations carried out.

H. Chater-Jack and A. J. Molloy, *Heart Trouble in the Family*, Health Horizon (for the Chest and Heart Association), 1970. Written by two medical social workers mainly for patients and their families, giving simple facts and advice about heart disease and a good picture of the social aspects of the problem.

Chest and Heart Association, *The Human Side of Heart Illness*, papers read at a two-day conference held in London in March 1970, Chest and Heart Association, 1970. Includes many aspects of heart disease, its prevention and management, with special references to the problems of maintaining normal life and work.

T. E. Gumpert, *Basic Cardiology*, 2nd edn, Wright, 1964. Really written for medical students, but with a simple approach which makes it suitable for nurses, at least for reference.

D. Longmore, *The Heart*, Wiedenfeld & Nicholson, 1971. Shows the importance of the heart in the working of the whole body. A description of the normal heart leads to its ills and their treatment and looks at future developments. All clearly and simply dealt with. Many illustrations.

M. Maclean and G. Scott, *Medical Treatment*, vol. 1, 3rd edn, Churchill Livingstone, 1968. Written for doctors, but chapters 1–4 give a clear description of cardiovascular diseases and modern trends in treatment which are suitable for nurses.

F. Pallett, *Circulatory System : Physiology and Pharmacology*, Butterworth, 1971. Simple description of the way the heart works and the effects of drugs on this.

L. Schneider, *Lifeline*, Macmillan, 1960. Chapter 1 gives a simple account of what the circulatory system is about. Intended for the interested layman.

G. Whitteridge, *William Harvey and the Circulation of the Blood*, Macdonald, 1971. An interesting and scholarly description of the state of knowledge in Harvey's time and the evolution of his ideas. For the inquiring nurse.

Chapter 1 The circulatory system
Books

J. H. Green, *Basic Clinical Physiology*, Oxford University Press, 1969. Not simple, but a clear explanation relating basic concepts of physiology to the clinical situation. Chapters 2, 3 and 15 particularly relevant.

D. F. Horrobin, *Essential Physiology*, Medical & Technical Publishing Co. Ltd, 1973. This aims at providing a thoughtful understanding of concepts (instead of dogmatic facts) from which each student can appreciate logically how and why things work in the body.

A. E. Hugh, *Cardiovascular System*, Butterworth, 1971. The presentation of anatomical facts is followed by summary paragraphs which constitute a test of material understood.

R. W. D. Turner, *Electrocardiography*, 3rd edn, Livingstone, 1969. Although written for doctors, the first chapter gives a straightforward explanation of how it is done and what it signifies.

Articles

C. Powell, 'Cardiograms for nurses', *Nursing Times*, vol. 66, 10 Sept. 1970, pp. 1157–79. A clear and simple introduction to the normal cardiogram and the way in which it is recorded.

Chapter 2 Heart failure
Books

H. Gibson, *Modern Medicine for Nurses*, Blackwell Scientific, 1972. Clear outline of the condition and factors leading to heart failure, with outline of clinical features and treatment.

G. R. Kelman, *Physiology : A Clinical Approach*, Churchill Livingstone, 1962. Written primarily for doctors, but should be at the level of an intelligent nurse. It links the action of the heart with the results of inefficient action in failure.

Articles

S. J. Hopkins, 'New drugs for old', *Nursing Times*, vol. 68, 6 July 1972, pp. 841–3. This gives the logical basis for the use of drugs, and the way in which they relieve heart failure.

G. Ismay 'Congestive cardiac failure', *Nursing Times*, vol. 68, 29 June 1972, pp. 797–800. How the heart fails and why. How it causes other organs to fail – with the resulting symptoms.

W. Melville Arnott, 'Heart failure', *British Medical Journal*, 1966, vol. 1, 25 June 1966, pp. 1585–8. Gives a clear description of the causes of heart failure and the effects of inadequate heart action on the body's activities, with outline of treatment.

Chapter 3 Ischaemic heart disease
Books

D. Cargill, *How to Avoid a Coronary Thrombosis*, Hamish Hamilton, 1967. A simple account of the heart and ischaemic heart disease, with a survey of causes and risks, leading to advice on how to avoid the disease.

N. L. Goodland, *Coronary Care*, Wright, 1970. A manual for nurses working with these patients, giving the nature of the condition, its effects and complications, with nursing care in hospital and at home – including the use of machines in a Coronary Care Unit.

P. J. Hubner, *Nurses' Guide to Cardiac Monitoring*, Baillière Tindall, 1971. Derived from lectures given to nurses in Coronary Care Units, it gives clear details of aims, methods, observations and machines.

E. R. Nye and P. G. Wood, *Exercise and the Coronary Patient*, Wolfe, 1971. A simple account of an exercise programme for patients recovering from heart attacks, introduced by anatomy and physiology of the coronary circulation. Intended for physiotherapists, but suitable for nurses.

L. Rose, *Coronary Wife*, Angus & Robertson, Sydney, 1972. A book that supplies helpful information and support to families of patients. Its discursive form covers much factual material.

Royal College of Nursing and National Council of Nurses of the United Kingdom, *Community Coronary Care*, report of conference in London, June 1971, Royal College of Nursing, 1971. Subjects include immediate care, family and patient support, long-term education and rehabilitation, the role of the nurse.

Articles

D. Christie, 'Prevention of heart attacks', *Physiotherapy*, vol. 58, October 1972, pp. 348–51. Factors predisposing to heart attack, showing how risk can be minimized by attention to these.

J. Clark, 'Heart disease – no. 1 killer', *Nursing Mirror*, vol. 135, 4 Aug. 1972, pp. 7–9. A survey of the problem of coronary disease today, with causes, prevention and speculation for the future.

G. S. Crockett, 'Patient monitoring', *Nursing Times*, vol. 66, 7 May 1970, pp. 581–3. An account of the usefulness of a monitoring system for patients with ischaemic heart disease, and the role of the nurse in connection with it.

R. A. Leach, 'Coronary thrombosis – a nursing care study', *Nursing Mirror*, vol. 136, 26 Jan. 1973, pp. 39–40. A straightforward description of the patient and treatment.

J. McCarthy, 'Cardiac arrest', *Nursing Times*, vol. 66, 10 Sept. 1970, p. 1178. A short and simple account by a pupil nurse of what happened when one of her patients suffered, and recovered from, a cardiac arrest.

H. C. Miller, 'Medical and surgical treatment of angina pectoris', *Physiotherapy*, vol. 58, October 1972, pp. 344–7. A simple exposition of the medical treatment of the disorder and its underlying condition, and an assessment of surgical treatment.

A. Morley and M. Spark, 'Resuscitation and the nurse', *Nursing Times*, vol. 66, 25 June 1970, pp. 814–5. Some methods of resuscitation and what the nurse needs to know about them.

P. G. F. Nixon, 'Rehabilitation of the coronary patient', *Physiotherapy*, vol. 58, October 1972, pp. 336–8. The principles underlying rehabilitation, and suggested methods.

S. F. Nunney, 'A patient with an inferior myocardial infarction', *Nursing Times*, vol. 68, 21 Sept. 1972, pp. 1178–80. A nursing care study of the patient, first in the Intensive Care Unit and then in the ward.

I. Robinson, 'Myocardial infarction – nursing case study', *Nursing Times*, vol. 68, 16 Nov. 1972, pp. 1442–5. Details of treatment and recovery, with helpful diagrams.

J. E. Robinson, 'Cardiac arrest and the nurse's duties', *Nursing Mirror*, vol. 136, 23 Feb. 1973, pp. 30–2. Some do's and don'ts – how to know that cardiac arrest has occurred and what the nurse should do about it.

T. Semple, 'Aftercare of heart attacks', *Rehabilitation*, no. 81, April/June 1972, pp. 21–3. A brief outline of the management of a patient after a heart attack, with advice to the patient's family.

D. Short and M. Stowers, 'Earliest symptoms of coronary heart disease and their recognition', *British Medical Journal*, vol. 2, 13 May 1972, pp. 387–91. A clear, though detailed, description of how to recognize this disease. Meant for doctors, but well at nurses' level.

Chapter 4 Abnormal rhythms and conduction
Books

J. Gibson, *Modern Medicine for Nurses*, 2nd edn, Blackwell, 1972. Chapter 3 gives a clear account of the conditions and the factors leading up to abnormal rhythms, with clinical features and a brief outline of treatment.

Articles

K. Dawson Butterworth, 'Heart block and the nurse's role in treatment', *Nursing Mirror*, vol. 124, 24 July 1967, pp. 372–4. A brief description of the condition, how it arises, its diagnosis and treatment, with special reference to the role of the nurse.

D. E. Foster, 'A patient with complete heart block', *Nursing Times*, vol. 63, 12 May 1967, pp. 616–18. A nursing care study of the patient treated first by 'drip' and then by implanting a cardiac pacemaker.

J. Geddes, 'Pacemakers keep some people ticking', *Nursing Times*, vol. 68, 6 Jan. 1972, pp. 5–8. Heart block and its control by pacemakers.

M. A. Martin, 'Cardiac arrhythmias', *British Journal of Clinical Practice*, vol. 26, March 1972, pp. 109–12. Although intended for doctors, this is a clear list of the different arrhythmias and their treatment, and could be of use to the nurse.

D. R. Redwood, 'Heart block and cardiac pacemakers', *Nursing Times*, vol. 63, 12 May 1967, pp. 614–16. Emergency and long-term treatment of heart block.

D. P. Siggens, 'The implanted cardiac pacemaker', *Nursing Times*, vol. 68, 23 March 1972, pp. 335–7. A description of the mechanism in the heart for making rhythmical contractions and how in heart block this can be replaced by an implanted electrical generator.

S. E. Smith, 'Drugs and the heart', *Nursing Times*, vol. 69, 16 March 1972, pp. 317–18. The use of digitalis, antiarhythmic agents and beta-receptor blockers in treating heart arrhythmias. A clear statement of facts.

C. Powell, 'Cardiograms for nurses', *Nursing Times*, vol. 66, 10 Sept. 1970, pp. 1157–9. A clear and simple introduction to the normal cardiogram and the way it is recorded.

C. Powell, 'Normal and abnormal rhythms', *Nursing Times*, vol. 66, 10 Sept. 1970, pp. 1202–4. A clear exposition of what makes the normal heart rhythm and some of the things which can go wrong with it.

C. Powell, 'Ventricular abnormal rhythms', *Nursing Times*, vol. 66, 24 Sept. 1970, pp. 1229–31. Some of the commoner abnormalities and how to recognize them.

C. Powell, 'The nurse, the patient, the machine', *Nursing Times*, vol. 66, 1 Oct. 1970, pp. 1267–70. The role of the nurse caring for a patient attached to some mechanical apparatus.

Chapter 5 High blood pressure
Books

G. Pickering, *Hypertension: Causes, Consequences and Management*, Churchill, 1970. A summary of the facts needed for understanding the condition and the problems of those who suffer from it.

Articles

A. Barham-Carter, 'Hypertension – its cause and treatment', *Nursing Times*, vol. 67, 6 May 1971, pp. 531–3. A short account of hypertension, its causes and possible treatment.

M. Hamilton, 'Management of hypertension', *Nursing Mirror*, vol. 132, 15 Jan. 1971, pp. 33–7. Different forms of treatment and the prevention of possible complications.

S. J. Hopkins, 'New drugs for old', *Nursing Times*, vol. 68, 6 July 1972, pp. 841–3. This gives the logical basis for the use of drugs and their value in treating hypertension.

Chapter 6 Heart valve disease
Books

R. G. Brackenridge, *Essential Medicine: A guide to Important Principles*, Medical & Technical Publishing Ltd, 1971. Chapter 4 gives a short classification of valvular heart disease with symptoms, signs and treatment.

J. C. Houston, C. L. Joiner and J. R. Trounce, *A Short Textbook of Medicine*, 4th edn, English Universities Press, 1972. Chapter 4 gives a clear account of rheumatic heart disease and the valvular disorders resulting from it.

A. R. Southwood, *Heart Disease: Some Ways to Prevent It*, Heinemann, 1962. Chapter 4 deals with rheumatic heart disease, its causes and prevention.

Articles

M. B. Bradby, 'Prosthetic valves in cardiac surgery 1: Valvular disease', *Nursing Times*, vol. 59, 19 July 1963, pp. 901–2. A short account of valvular disease.

M. B. Bradby, 'Prosthetic valves in cardiac surgery 2: Valvular supply', *Nursing Times*, vol. 59, 26 July 1962, 926–8. An account of the different types of operation and the post-operative management.

P. J. D. Ennis, 'A patient with aortic valve incompetence', *Nursing Times*, vol. 69, 7 June 1973, pp. 733–5. A nursing case study of a young man who had an operation for aortic valve replacement. Gives investigations carried out and pre- and post-operative care, as well as a description of the actual operation.

R. Gilbait, 'Heart valve replacement', *Nursing Times*, vol. 68, 16 Nov. 1972, pp. 1439–41. A detailed description of the various operations and the responsibilities of the theatre nurse.

Chapter 7 Congenital heart disease
Books

M. A. Duncombe, *Aids to Paediatric Nursing*, 3rd edn, Baillière Tindall, 1969, pp. 169–86. Chapter 10 deals with the cardiovascular system and gives a simple description of the congenital abnormalities, their treatment, and the care of babies with these conditions.

L. Schamroth and F. Segal, *An Introduction to Congenital Heart Disease*, Blackwell, 1960. Although written for doctors, this is a useful reference book for nurses, giving clear line drawings of abnormalities and discussing their treatment.

Articles

I. Andrews, 'Correction of atrial septal defect in a child', *Nursing Times*, vol. 69 22 Feb. 1973, pp. 238–40. A nursing care study giving details of pre- and post-operative care, as well as an account of the operation.

E. M. George, 'Care of children undergoing cardiac surgery', *Nursing Times*, vol. 68, 13 Sept. 1972, pp. 39–41. An experienced Ward Sister describes the special care a child needs.

T. Hamilton, 'Major open heart surgery in childhood', *Nursing Times*, vol. 68, 20 Jan. 1972, pp. 70–6. An account of detailed and careful nursing care of a child having heart surgery (for atrial septal defect), with description of heart-lung machine.

D. Laycock, 'Waterston's operation for Fallot's tetralogy', *Nursing Times*, vol. 68, 25 May 1968, pp. 632–4. A nursing care study of a little boy of $2\frac{1}{2}$ who had correction of his congenital heart lesion. The operation and his nursing care are described in detail.

F. Mantle, 'Total correction of Fallot's tetralogy and patent foramen ovale', *Nursing Times*, vol. 68, 27 July 1972, pp. 934–6. Nursing care study of a little boy, showing the treatment and care he received leading to good recovery.

Chapter 8 The lungs and pulmonary circulation in heart disease
Books

J. Gibson, *Modern Medicine for Nurses*, Blackwell, 1972. Chapter 3 gives a clear account of the conditions and the factors leading to them, with clinical features and a brief outline of treatment.

Articles

A. G. Chappell, 'Pulmonary embolism', *Nursing Mirror*, vol. 132, 8 Jan. 1971, pp. 26–8. An account of the causes, clinical features, diagnosis, treatment and prevention of this condition.

C. Illingworth, 'Post-operative thrombosis and pulmonary embolism', *Nursing Times*, vol. 66, 9 April 1970, pp. 459–60. The effect of surgery on blood clotting and the nurse's role in prevention, and the observation of signs of onset of the conditions.

L. Reid, 'Cor pulmonale', *Nursing Mirror*, vol. 136, 1 June 1973, pp. 26–7. The conditions leading to this and how they produce it, with a brief outline of treatment and observations.

S. Stock, 'Preventing pulmonary embolism', *New Scientist*, vol. 56, 26 Oct. 1972, pp. 202–4. An account of the factors causing thrombosis and embolism, with principles of treatment and prevention.

Chapter 9 Pericardial, myocardial and endocardial disease
Books

R. G. Brackenridge, *Essential Medicine*, Medical *&* Technical Publishing Co. Ltd, 1971. Chapter 4 gives a short account of endocarditis, pericarditis and myocarditis, cardiomyopathy, with signs and symptoms, causes, treatment and prevention.

Chapter 10 Diseases of arteries and veins
Books

G. Fegan, *Varicose Veins : Compression Sclerotherapy*, Heinemann, 1967. A comprehensive study of the subject, showing how patients can be successfully treated without admission to hospital or loss of work time.

R. R. Foot, *The Physical Treatment of Varicose Ulcers : A Practical Manual for the Physiotherapist and Nurse*, Livingstone, 1958. A small book giving a clear outline of the anatomy of the venous system, the causes of varicose ulcers, general treatment and aftercare – with special reference to the role of the nurse aud physiotherapist.

J. Gibson, *Modern Medicine for Nurses*, Blackwell, 1972. Clear, concise account of the conditions, causes, clinical features and treatment.

J. A. Gillespie and D. M. Douglas, *Some Aspects of Obliterative Vascular Disease of the Lower Limb*, Livingstone, 1961. Although written for doctors, this book gives a clear account of the causes and effects of arterial disease, with some of the measures used to combat and alleviate it. Chapters 1, 2 and 11 are relevant for nurses.

A. J. H. Raine, *Arterial Surgery for Nurses*, Macmillan (for *Nursing Times*), 1965. A series of articles describing conditions for which surgery is carried out, the operations performed and post-operative care, and palliative measures where surgery is inadvisable.

S. L. Rivlin, *A New Way with Old Leg Ulcers : A Practical and Illustrated Manual for Nurses*, Pitman Medical, 1963. A simple yet detailed manual dealing with the treatment of chronic leg ulcers, with special reference to causes. Written for nurses in the community.

C. R. Savage, *Vascular Surgery*, Pitman, 1970. A detailed and comprehensive account of vascular disease and its treatment, both conservative and surgical.

Articles

G. M. Grown, 'Case study – varicose vein', *District Nursing*, vol. 15, June 1972, pp. 59–60. An account of the treatment and progress of a patient with a varicose vein nursed at home.

D. P. Burkitt, 'Varicose veins, deep vein thrombosis and haemorrhoids', *British Medical Journal*, vol. 2, 3 June 1972, pp. 556–61. Some new ideas on the causes of these conditions.

A. G. Chappell, 'Pulmonary embolism', *Nursing Mirror*, vol. 132, 8 Jan. 1971, pp. 26–8. An account of the causes, clinical features, diagnosis, treatment and prevention of this condition.

A. M. Davies, 'Nursing care study, streptokinase therapy for deep vein thrombosis', *Nursing Times*, vol. 69, 15 Feb. 1973, pp. 211–12. The uses of streptokinase are described, together with its dangers and effects on the patient.

H. Dodd, 'Varicose veins and venous disorders of the lower limbs 1', *Nursing Mirror*, vol. 135, 17 Nov. 1972, pp. 42–7. Anatomy and physiology of the veins of the lower limbs. The mechanics of varicose veins, their causes and complications.

H. Dodd, 'Varicose veins and venous disorders of the lower limbs 2', *Nursing Mirror*, vol. 135, 24 Nov. 1972, pp. 46–51. Methods of diagnosis and all the different forms of surgical treatment.

H. Ellis, 'Arteriosclerotic disease of the lower limbs', *Nursing Times*, vol. 69, 31 May 1973, pp. 698–700. This gives the clinical features of the disease, in the elderly, the predisposing factors and some of the modern forms of treatment.

R. H. Harvey, 'Nursing care in direct arterial surgery', *Nursing Times*, vol. 63, 11 Aug. 1963, pp. 1055–6. The pre- and post-operative care of patients having arterial surgery.

N. H. Hills and J. S. Calnan, 'Deep vein thrombosis after surgery', *Nursing Mirror*, vol. 135, 21 July 1972, pp. 29–30. This gives a clear account of the causes, treatment and prevention of this condition.

C. Illingworth, 'Vascular diseases of the lower limbs', *Nursing Times*, vol. 66, 7 May 1970, pp. 591–2. An account of their onset, conservative and surgical treatment, and the importance of preventive measures.

M. Martin, 'Traumatic rupture of aorta', *Nursing Times*, vol. 65, 14 Aug. 1969, pp. 1031–4. The story of a man who survived rupture of the aorta in a road accident. How he was treated and cared for until convalescence.

P. F. Meyer, 'Arteriosclerosis', *Nursing Mirror*, vol. 127, 29 Nov. 1968, pp. 28–32. An account of how it arises and what it does to the body.

D. J. Rhodes and G. J. Hadfield, 'Treatment of varicose veins', *Practitioner*, vol. 208, June 1972, pp. 809–15. Showing how injection and compression are frequently successful, the patient remaining ambulant and usually at risk during treatment.

C. R. Savage, 'Direct arterial surgery', *Nursing Times*, vol. 63, 11 Aug. 1967, pp. 1052–5. Some of the conditions for which surgery is indicated and the operations performed to relieve them.

N. Vukovitch, 'A clinic for varicose veins', *Nursing Times*, vol. 68, 31 Aug. 1972, pp. 1090–2. A description of the methods used successfully in the author's clinic.

T. G. Wadsworth, 'Post-operative deep vein thrombosis', *Nursing Mirror*, vol. 134, 28 Jan. 1972, pp. 28–30. Common causes and some suggestions for prevention.

W. F. Walker, 'Atherosclerosis', *Physiotherapy*, vol. 58, October 1972, pp. 328–31. A comprehensive review of what this is, predisposing factors, clinical effects and management.

Acknowledgements

We wish to thank the following for permission to use material that has been the basis for some of the illustrations.

For Figures 8 and 15: W. B. Saunders Company, *Cardiovascular Dynamics* (3rd edn) by Robert F. Rushmer. For Figure 13: Heinemann Medical Books Ltd, *Modern Urology for Nurses* (2nd edn), by James O. Robinson. For Figures 22 and 55: Blackwell Scientific Publications, *Medical and Surgical Cardiology* by W. Cleland *et al.* For Figure 25: Butterworth & Co., *Coronary Care Units* by W. J. Grace and V. Keyloun. For Figure 27: Heinemann Medical Books Ltd, *Cardio-Respiratory Resuscitation* by A. Gilston and L. Resnekov. For Figure 36: Bailliere Tindall, *Cardiology* by D. G. Julian. For Figure 37: Blackwell Scientific Publications, *An Introduction to Electrocardiography* (3rd edn) by L. Shamroth. For Figures 46 and 47: Churchill Livingstone, *Auscultation of the Heart and Phonocardiography* by A. Leatham. For Figures 44 and 45: Orbis Publishing Company, *Mind and Body*. For Figures 57, 60, 72, 75, 76, 94 and 95: Blackwell Scientific Publications, *Lecture Notes on Cardiology* by J. S. Fleming and M. V. Braimbridge. For Figure 61: Macmillan, London and Basingstoke, *Textbook of Human Anatomy* by W. J. Hamilton. For Figures 64 and 84: Aldus Books Ltd, *Machines in Medicine* by Donald Longmore.

Figures 18, 23, 25, 28, 29, 30, 31, 33, 43, 52, 71 and 79: photographs by Peter G. Tucker. Figures 50, 66, 67 and 68: X-rays courtesy Edgware General Hospital. Figures 59, 70, 81 and 83: X-rays courtesy Hammersmith Hospital. Figure 88: courtesy Dr Celia Oakley.

Index